ARKANA

Therapeutic Touch

Janet Macrae, PhD, RN, has taught more than two hundred
Therapeutic Touch workshops in nursing schools and healing
centres in the United States. She was head nurse of a paediatric
unit at Columbia Presbyterian Medical Center in New York City
from 1973 to 1975, and from 1982 to 1987 was an adjunct
assistant professor in the Division of Nursing at New York
University. Since 1981 she has had a private practice in
Therapeutic Touch in New York City.

Therapeutic Touch
A Practical Guide

Janet Macrae

with illustrations by Michael Sellon

ARKANA

ARKANA

Published by the Penguin Group
Penguin Books Ltd, 27 Wrights Lane, London W8 5TZ, England
Penguin Books USA Inc., 375 Hudson Street, New York, New York 10014, USA
Penguin Books Australia Ltd, Ringwood, Victoria, Australia
Penguin Books Canada Ltd, 10 Alcorn Avenue, Toronto, Ontario, Canada M4V 3B2
Penguin Books (NZ) Ltd, 182–190 Wairau Road, Auckland 10, New Zealand

Penguin Books Ltd, Registered Offices: Harmondsworth, Middlesex, England

First published in the USA by Alfred A. Knopf, Inc. 1988
and simultaneously in Canada by Random House of Canada Ltd
Published by Arkana 1990
3 5 7 9 10 8 6 4 2

NOTE TO READERS
The technique of Therapeutic Touch described in this book
is intended not as a substitute for medical treatment or
surgery but as a complement to them.

Printed in England by Clays Ltd, St Ives plc

*This book is dedicated to
Dora Kunz and Dee Krieger,
and to all my friends and colleagues
with whom I have been privileged
to share this healing journey.*

Contents

Contents

List of Diagrams and Charts

Preface

This book is a guide for the practice of Therapeutic Touch, which is a way of acting as an instrument of healing. The term "healing," in this context, refers to the integrating tendency within the individual as a whole: body, mind, and creative spirit, and so the focus is on the process of balancing the energies of the total person rather than on the treatment of specific physical diseases. Since the ability to assist the healing process through Therapeutic Touch is thought to be present in everyone, this book is addressed not only to health professionals but to anyone who would like to learn.

As I will discuss later, the main requirements on the part of the student are good health, compassion, and a willingness to discipline oneself and learn the basic aspects of the method. A sense of adventure is also helpful, because the practice of Therapeutic Touch involves opening oneself to a new dimension or mode of perceiving. Most of our knowledge of the world comes through our physical senses or their extensions by way of instruments such as microscopes and telescopes. We describe objects and events by the way they look, feel, sound, smell, and taste. The practice of Therapeutic Touch, however, is based on the concept of a subtle, *non-physical* energy, which sustains all living organisms. This energy is not an abstraction but a vitalizing, universal force, which is always present and available. The practice of Therapeutic Touch represents a conscious effort to draw upon this universal life energy and direct its flow for healing. I have tried to describe, as accurately as possible, how to attune to this subtle energy, identify various ways in which it can become disordered by disease, and help re-establish a normal flow. Since there are no adjectives in our language that directly pertain to subtle energy qualities, my descriptions should not be taken literally but should be regarded as analogies or metaphors. Thus when I say that a certain type of imbalance feels hot, I am not referring to the sensation of physical heat, which we feel with the receptors in our skin. Rather, I am trying to describe an energy quality that has a feeling-tone resembling heat. As these subtle cues are perceived subjectively and thus can be described in slightly different ways, I often use several adjectives — at the risk of appearing redundant — to help clarify my meaning.

Chapter 1 contains a general introduction to Therapeutic Touch, based on those questions that are most frequently asked during lectures and demonstrations. In Chapter 2 I have explained the basic principles that

underlie the technique. Therapeutic Touch is an embodi-
ment of these fundamental ideas and without them the
practice remains shallow and incomplete. In Chapter 3
I have outlined the method; but to avoid cluttering it
with details, I have saved a discussion of various issues
and problems (all of which have been raised by students)
for the chapter that follows it. And finally, since the
practice of Therapeutic Touch involves making oneself
an instrument for the healing force, the last chapter is
concerned with the transformation of the practitioner.
One *becomes,* so to speak, what one has learned.

Since English does not have one pronoun for both
sexes, I have used "he" and "she" interchangeably instead
of the cumbersome "he/she" construction, for I wanted
the words to flow in a dance that would reflect, in some
measure, the beauty of this method of healing. I have
used the word "patient" instead of "healee" or "client"
simply because this is the term with which I am most
familiar and comfortable as a nurse with a traditional
education. I have avoided using the word "healer" in
reference to the individual who is practicing Therapeutic Touch because I feel this term can be very misleading.
There is no simple answer to the question "Who is
doing the healing?" Is it the innate healing potential
within all living things? Is it the life energy, a universal
force that has order as its basis? Is it the practitioner,
who serves as a conduit or an instrument? Or is it a
combination of all three at a crucial moment?[1] I have
tried to explain what I understand about assisting the
healing process through Therapeutic Touch, but essentially it remains a mystery, as does life itself.

I have focused on the use of Therapeutic Touch
with human beings because most of my experience with

Therapeutic Touch

A Practical Guide

1

An Introduction to Therapeutic Touch

Nature alone cures.... And what nursing has to do ... is to put the patient in the best condition for nature to act upon him.

FLORENCE NIGHTINGALE, *Notes on Nursing*

Therapeutic Touch has been derived from the ancient practice of the laying-on of hands. It is based on the fundamental assumption that there is a universal life energy that sustains all living organisms. Although the idea of a subtle vital energy is only just beginning to be accepted in Western medicine, it has long been a feature of Eastern therapeutic systems. In India, for example, the energy is called *prana* and is associated with the breath. From ancient times, breathing exercises known as *pranayama* (literally translated as the "regulation of prana") were designed to enhance well-being through a balancing of the life-energy flow.

Currently, the concept of a universal life energy is being linked to field theory and seen as exhibiting the characteristics of a force field.[3] In physical science, a field is generally defined as a continuous quality or condition throughout space. For example, we know that gravity, as a field, exists everywhere in space; it is more intense, however, in the area around a planet or other celestial body. Since life is "an inherent principle in the dynamics of the universe,"[4] we make the assumption that the vital energy is also a field force, that is, that it permeates space, becoming more concentrated within and around living organisms. Thus all living things without exception share in a generalized life-energy field, in the same way that all physical objects in space are subject to gravity.

In a state of health, the life energy flows freely in, through, and out of the organism in a balanced manner, nourishing all the organs of the body. In disease, the flow of the energy is obstructed, disordered, and/or depleted. Therapeutic Touch practitioners, having learned to attune to the universal field through a conscious intent, direct the life energy into the patients to enhance their vitality. The practitioners also help the patients assimilate the energy by releasing congestion and balancing areas where the flow has become disordered. Drawing upon the universal field, the practitioners do not become drained of their own energy but, on the contrary, are continually replenished. Since the localized field of the patient penetrates and extends beyond the body, actual physical contact is not necessary for Therapeutic Touch. In fact, for reasons that will be discussed later, most practitioners prefer to work a few inches from the surface of the patient's skin.

Although Therapeutic Touch is a new technique in our present health care system, it appears to be timeless and universal. I remember, as a beginning practitioner, treating a little boy who was in the hospital dying of cancer. The child's grandfather, who spoke very little English, would visit sometimes, but as it was so difficult for him to see the boy in this condition, he would usually withdraw and sit looking out the window. As soon as I started to use Therapeutic Touch, however, the grandfather came immediately to the bedside and joined me in the practice. He knew exactly what to do and we worked together, beautifully synchronized, in silence. When I felt that the boy had had enough, I looked at his grandfather: our eyes met, he nodded and then went back to the window. I knew then that Therapeutic Touch is a mode of communication in its own right. It is the same art the world over, needing, like music, no interpretation.

In the United States the person principally responsible for the contemporary reintroduction and development of this technique is Dora Kunz, a highly gifted therapist. She hypothesized that the ability to assist healing, in a manner such as the laying-on of hands, is not a talent bestowed on special individuals but a capacity innate in all human beings. From careful observations of the work of many well-known healers, she defined the principles and goals of an approach that she felt had universal application and could be taught to those with a genuine interest. Dr. Dolores Krieger participated in the development of this approach and it was she who gave it the name Therapeutic Touch.[5] Since the early 1970s, the technique has been refined and its effects documented by many practitioners. This refinement process is far from complete, however, for if Therapeutic Touch is truly an aspect of our human potential its possibilities for further development are limitless.

Therapeutic Touch

In 1975, the *American Journal of Nursing* published an experiment conducted by Dr. Krieger, which demonstrated a significantly greater increase in the mean hemoglobin level of a group of patients who received Therapeutic Touch than in that of a control group of patients who received routine nursing care.[6] For several reasons, this experiment was a milestone in the development of Therapeutic Touch into a recognized clinical method.

First of all, it was conducted in New York City hospitals, thus setting an important precedent. Although Therapeutic Touch was a somewhat unorthodox procedure, it began to be integrated into our traditional health care system. Most of my workshops, and those of my colleagues as well, are conducted in hospitals and nursing schools. We look upon Therapeutic Touch as complementary to medical and surgical procedures—not as a substitute for them.

Second, registered nurses with no previous experience in this type of healing participated in the experiment, thus supporting the view that Therapeutic Touch is a latent capacity within all human beings. I find that most people who attend the workshops can learn the basics quickly, but—as with any skill—their ability improves with practice.

Finally, the experiment indicated that it is indeed possible to gain knowledge about Therapeutic Touch through the use of controlled methods of scientific research. Although this technique requires a particularly subjective state on the part of the practitioner, it is nevertheless a consciously controlled state and can therefore be approached scientifically. At the same time, however, this healing method requires a level of sensitivity and skill that elevates it to the status of an art.

6

My colleagues and I have found that Therapeutic Touch is particularly helpful for people who are suffering from wounds and infections, from those at home with minor cuts and burns or the common cold to those in the hospital recuperating from surgery. The method not only helps to alleviate discomfort but also tends to speed up the healing process. Theoretically, this could be expected because directing life energy (or healing energy, as it is sometimes called) to a patient should be strengthening and thus foster a quicker recovery. These clinical observations are consistent with the findings of a carefully designed series of experiments in which there was a significant increase in the rate of wound healing in mice who received the laying-on of hands, a related procedure.[7]

As is the case with any method of treatment, people respond in their own way to Therapeutic Touch. This is true even among those with the same type of problem. One evening, for instance, I treated three school-age boys who were admitted to the hospital with acute asthmatic attacks. The first boy stopped wheezing immediately afterwards; the second boy's condition did not improve at all; and while the third boy continued to wheeze, his breathing became much easier and he fell asleep. Sometimes a person with several ailments will find that each one responds differently to Therapeutic Touch. One man, after his first treatment, said that his asthmatic condition was unchanged but that a rash which had been bothering him for weeks had disappeared almost immediately.

Sometimes a person responds psychologically more than physically. After a treatment the patient may say, for example, "I still have my pain but it doesn't bother me so much right now." I once treated a woman who was to have surgery for bowel cancer the following week. At one point I felt an energy shift, which was accompanied by a profound feeling of peace. Afterwards, she said, "I saw the IVs, the tubes, the drains—everything I have to face—and all my fear left me." This woman's experience is also a good illustration of the fact that the process of healing, that is, restoring wholeness, means helping each patient open up and tap, so to speak, an inner reservoir of peace, insight, and strength that is available to all.

We have found that the effectiveness of Therapeutic Touch is not dependent on the recipient's conscious belief, as is the case with faith healing. All that is required on the part of an ill person is simply to sit or lie down quietly for about fifteen to twenty minutes while someone gives the treatment. I have used Therapeutic Touch to help babies and toddlers, who certainly could not profess any faith in the method, and teenagers who were often quite skeptical. The mouse experiments mentioned above are another indication that conscious belief is not necessary for beneficial results. Interestingly enough, the reverse can and does happen. People have sometimes come to me for treatments in the firm belief that Therapeutic Touch would help them, only to find that very little improvement occurred. In view of the current research in biofeedback and in the placebo effect, which demonstrates that the quality of a person's thoughts can have a measurable effect on his body, it is reasonable to suppose that the degree to which a person believes in the efficacy of Therapeutic Touch should affect, to some extent, the outcome of the treatment. In view of the above observations, however, it is certain that there are other factors besides conscious belief that influence one's response to the healing process.

In general, a person with an acute illness responds more quickly to Therapeutic Touch than does one with a chronic illness. If a healthy person has a bout of indigestion after a holiday party, this can usually be relieved after one treatment, whereas a person with a chronic gastrointestinal problem would probably need regular treatments over an extended period of time. When a person has been ill for many years, the disabling energy pattern becomes "set" or ingrained. During the healing process we try to help a person retrain the energy flow—to establish new habit patterns, so to speak, which are more open and balanced. Just as an athletic training program requires consistent practice with appropriate help and feedback from a coach, so also does a healing or energy-balancing program. For example, the condition of a woman with severe emphysema (which she had had for at least twenty years) improved gradually at first, but then suddenly—after eight months of weekly treatments—a fairly dramatic change began to occur. Her breathing became easier, she could walk briskly again, and her writing ability, which she felt she had lost, spontaneously returned. This woman's experience illustrates not only the cumulative effect of regular Therapeutic Touch treatments but also the fact that the most profound healing generally involves a psychological as well as a physical change.

Very often we are unaware of the mental and emotional aspects of a physical problem.

When we are under stress—or if we know that we will be under stress—we do not necessarily associate it with the moment. Very often we unconsciously go back into our memories and react to the stress of the past and not to the experience of the present. Part of that may be based on reality but part may be blown all out of proportion. If the memory holds onto painful experiences, it leads to disease.[8]

Effective healing, therefore, often necessitates an insight into one's psychological patterns together with a willingness to change them. For example, sometimes a person has a physical problem that is associated with, and/or aggravated by, feelings of resentment toward some person or situation. Unless he realizes this connection and can drop the resentment, there may be only a superficial healing—that is, a temporary relief of physical symptoms. In view of this, we can say that an individual's *habitual and/or unconscious thinking and feeling patterns* affect the outcome of the treatment much more than does his faith or belief in the power of Therapeutic Touch.

One way in which this method helps to bring about a more profound healing is through evoking a state of relaxation in which the individual is centered in the present moment. In such a state it becomes easier to diminish negative patterns established in the past.[9] During a treatment, one can generally see the common signs of relaxation in the patient, such as slower and deeper breathing, a loosening of muscle tension, and the dilation of peripheral blood vessels, which makes the hands and feet warm up and the face flush. Indeed, when Therapeutic Touch was first being developed, such observable signs of relaxation were the first indications that the method was effective.[10] These observations were later documented in a case study in which three subjects were monitored physiologically during Therapeutic Touch.[11] The recordings of the subjects' brain waves, muscle tension, skin conductance, temperature, and heart rate all indicated that they were in a deeply relaxed state. Afterwards, the subjects confirmed the physiological data by reporting that during the treatment, they had felt relaxed and in a state of well-being.

Two subsequent experiments measured the effects of Therapeutic Touch on the acute anxiety of hospitalized cardiovascular patients.[12, 13] It was thought that if Therapeutic Touch was able to induce a state of physical relaxation, it might also be able to reduce the anxiety often associated with physical tension. The patients' anxiety levels were measured on a standardized self-evaluation questionnaire before and after treatment, and the results of both experiments were similar: the mean post-test anxiety scores of the Therapeutic Touch groups were significantly lower than those of the control groups.

Because Therapeutic Touch helps to reduce anxiety we have found it to be helpful not only for people with stress-related physical disorders, such as tension headaches,[14] high blood pressure, and ulcers, but also for those undergoing an emotional crisis. It is becoming apparent that the process has an integrating as well as a calming effect. A person who comes for a treatment in an upset state of mind will often say afterwards, "I feel more together," or "I feel less scattered," or "I feel like myself again." This fact is important because if unresolved emotional conflict (such as negative memory patterns) can lead to physical disease, then Therapeutic Touch—given during the time of a crisis—could help prevent the emergence of subsequent disorders. This method, therefore, can be used as a helpful adjunct to psychotherapy as well as to medical and surgical treatment. It can also be used very effectively at home, when a friend or family member is tired and upset.

Since words are not necessary for Therapeutic Touch, the treatment can be a way of communicating with the terminally ill, who are often too tired to speak. Just because someone is very near death does not mean that he cannot benefit from this method; in fact, my colleagues and I have found that the terminally ill are often very responsive to the healing process.

> We . . . have to come to grips with the fact that the outcome of many diseases is death. If one can accept this and help a person through compassion in any way to reduce pain and to die peacefully, that is also a kind of healing. [15]

From the perspective of Therapeutic Touch, the physical body is only one aspect of our total being; thus it is possible to be "healed" without necessarily being "cured" of a specific disease. The focus of this method is on a broad concept of healing based on the balance of energy flow within the individual as a whole—and this whole includes body, mind, and inner spirit. The effectiveness of a treatment, therefore, can be evaluated only in relation to the total well-being of the individual patient.

As mentioned earlier, Therapeutic Touch is considered by those who practice it to be a capacity present in all human beings—a seed, so to speak, that lies within us all. Cultivating the seed requires three things: good health, compassion, and discipline. *Good health* implies a basic sense of wholeness, or a general feeling of well-being. *Compassion* is the ability to empathize with those who are suffering; it implies a desire to help others without any other motivation or personal aim. The action is its own reward. Compassion, therefore, should never be confused with a state of emotional attachment or personal investment, for such attitudes actually hinder the healing process. Some *self-discipline* is necessary because Therapeutic Touch is a highly refined skill that is developed through regular practice. It is true that one can help people immediately after learning the basics (a fact that amazes many beginners), but with some dedicated practice one's work becomes deeper and much more effective. This does not imply a dreary apprenticeship, however, because working with Therapeutic Touch is always interesting and full of surprises. A student who had been giving treatments for a few months said, in a very matter-of-fact way, "This has improved the quality of my life." All of us who are involved with Therapeutic Touch would agree with her and it is my hope that, as you learn this method, you also will find that it reveals an entirely new dimension of meaning and experience.

2

The Guiding Principles

Before learning the basic skills of Therapeutic Touch, you must understand the fundamental principles upon which the method is based. The verb "to heal" comes from the Anglo-Saxon word *hǣlan,* which means "to make whole." We know from a study of biological science that living organisms are self-organizing wholes; through a continual interchange with the environment they are able to grow, develop, and maintain, restore, and reproduce themselves. The ability to heal, or to restore wholeness, is thus an innate capacity or tendency in all living things.

The concept of wholeness in turn implies the qualities of order and integrity. A "whole" is generally defined as a unified entity, a system, or a complete organization. Living organisms are dynamic self-organizing wholes in which the parts tend to function together in an orderly manner. The integrating or ordering principle seems, in a sense, to be even more fundamental than the individual organs and bodily systems, because if a part is damaged the organism has the ability to heal or restore the dynamic order of the whole. In fact, healing could be described as the intrinsic movement toward order within living organisms. We must always remember that the part can be healed only within the context of the whole. A branch cut from a tree withers and dies, but the living tree not only survives but can restore its essential symmetry and integrity.

From the point of view of Therapeutic Touch, disease is a form of disorder both within the individual and between the individual and the environment. The practitioner helps to reorder the patient's energy flow pattern, thus enhancing her innate drive toward wholeness. In Therapeutic Touch workshops, students sometimes comment that the idea of a tendency toward order within living organisms contradicts the second law of thermodynamics, which states that energy systems move toward greater disorder (entropy). This law, however, applies only to non-living and/or man-made systems, such as machines. A machine is a closed system that uses up energy; if this is not replenished by an outside agency the system will run down until it stops—a condition of maximum entropy. Living systems, on the other hand, are open, able to maintain their proper form and function through self-renewal by importing free energy from the environment. The flow of life is often described as being "negentropic," that is, contrary to entropy, evolving toward greater complexity of organization.[16] It is this negentropic thrust, or tendency, within the organism that is assisted through Therapeutic Touch.

The self-regulation by means of which living organisms grow and develop is accomplished through a continual exchange with the environment on many levels. Human beings, for example, partake of all the physical elements: earth, water, air, and fire (sunlight). We swim in a sea of living energy that interpenetrates and activates all our systems, from the simple to the more complex. Paradoxically, even though all living creatures are self-organizing and autonomous, they are completely dependent on this environmental interchange. In some mysterious way, living things are always changing and yet always the same; by participating in the universal flow of Nature they maintain their essential identity and integrity.

If life is characterized by an interchange of various qualities of energy, it can be assumed that any form of obstruction — either within the organism or between the organism and the environment — is contrary to Nature's tendencies and therefore unhealthy. We can find many physical examples of this fact: blockages in the respiratory system, the digestive system, the urinary system, and the circulatory system are all associated with ill health. When you learn Therapeutic Touch, you will discover that obstructions in the flow of the life energy also result in a diminution of well-being. We know that mental and emotional blockages not only hinder mature development but also lead to physical disease. On any level obstructions fragment the wholeness of the individual.

In order to help the ill person, the practitioner — whether orthodox or unorthodox — tries to remove the blockages so that the natural healing process can proceed more effectively. When an obstruction is removed from the lungs, for example, the patient is able to absorb more oxygen, which revitalizes all the tissues of the body. Similarly, when congestion of the vital energy is removed during a Therapeutic Touch treatment, the patient is able to absorb more energy from the environment and assimilate it more efficiently and thoroughly.

In addition to removing obstructions and balancing disorder, the practitioner directs the life energy into the ill person. This serves to strengthen the individual so that healing can occur more effectively. The concept of the energy field is essential with respect to this process, because it permits us to draw upon a larger, almost limitless resource for healing. If you were to think of yourself and the patient as separate buckets, one emptying its contents into the other, the donor would soon become depleted. If, on the other hand, you consciously draw from the universal field, you will be continually replenished from an inexhaustible source.

Within the context of Therapeutic Touch, human beings begin to take on a new and different guise. Instead of being solid entities that process various forms of energy from the environment, we perceive that they actually *are* the energy that they are processing. Dora Kunz and Erik Peper, working on a theory first proposed by F. L. Kunz,[17] use the concept of a field to describe not only physical and vital energies but *every human function,* including emotion, thought, and intuition. The emotional energy field, for example, permeates space but is more concentrated within and around living things. These concentrations, or localized individual fields, are characterized by the quality of the individual's emotions at any given moment. Emotions are thus not produced by the physical body and contained therein but are actually radiating patterns of energy that, traversing the universal field, continually influence the fields of others in the environment. This is the reason we can often "feel" someone's love or anger even when it has not been expressed in words. Our thinking patterns, also, are energies that emanate from us and are continually being picked up by others in our environment.

A human being is thus a localized interaction pattern within various universal fields of energy.

> This focus of energy is what we experience as *ourselves*. The different fields of an individual [i.e., the physical, vital, emotional, mental, and intuitional] can be perceived in terms of sub-categories related to specific functions. Somewhat analogous is the way white light can be perceived as a composite of all the colors, yet can be separated into its component spectral colors with the use of a prism.[18]

Body, mind, and spirit, therefore, are not separate substances or categories, but rather different energy frequencies that are continually interacting. A human being is a complex, multidimensional energy system. From this point of view, health or wholeness implies an inner balance among these different levels or dimensions of energy as well as an open, harmonious interchange between the individual and the environment.

The practice of Therapeutic Touch involves the use of oneself (that is, one's own localized energy field) as an instrument to help rebalance areas within the patient's field that have become obstructed and disordered by disease. As a relaxed, "totally present" state of being is required to do this, the practitioner has to have some control over his thoughts and emotions as well as his physical gestures. The use of conscious intent (sometimes called intentionality) is thus essential for the practice of Therapeutic Touch. The practitioner must establish the intent to become a calm, focused conduit for the universal life energy and to direct the energy to the patient. Biofeedback, with which most people are probably more familiar, is another healing method that requires the use of intentionality. During a biofeedback session, the individual establishes the intent to quiet and focus his mind, and since his mind influences his body, the monitors will indicate a relaxation response. Since the Therapeutic Touch practitioner is transferring energy through the universal field, however, his intent affects not only his own body, as in biofeedback, but also that of the patient.

This principle—that the life energy follows our intent—is clearly illustrated in one of the anxiety experiments mentioned previously.[19] In this study, the experimental group of patients received Therapeutic Touch from an experienced practitioner while the control group received a mimic treatment from a nurse who had not been taught the method. When delivering the treatments, both avoided physical contact, keeping their hands four to six inches from the surface of the patients' skin. The gestures were so similar that objective observers, watching them on videotape, could not tell the difference between Therapeutic Touch and the mimic treatment. The significant difference in anxiety reduction between the two groups thus supports the hypothesis that the effects of Therapeutic Touch are due to the practitioner's intent to direct energy to the patients.

It should be emphasized that intentionality is not emotion or personal desire but the much deeper force by means of which we mobilize and focus ourselves — mind and body — to carry out a specific purpose. In the case of Therapeutic Touch the purpose is to become an instrument of healing and to help living organisms restore their wholeness. As we discussed before, the ability to heal is characteristic of life, and life is an intrinsic aspect of the wholeness of nature. When an organism becomes ill, the innate drive to re-establish order is immediately mobilized. Nature, so to speak, acts with a purpose; so when we cooperate with nature by assisting the healing process we can say that our intent and nature's intent are in harmony.

If it is to be effective, the practice of Therapeutic Touch requires both compassion and integrity — a sense of the unity of all life and also a sense of our own wholeness. These qualities are not mutually exclusive; on the contrary, as you learn the method, you will see that they are mutually reinforcing. When we open ourselves in empathy and compassion to the ill person we establish an intense energy field interaction which is characteristic of Therapeutic Touch. However, unless we are also able to maintain our sense of wholeness or inner identity we can easily get "caught up" in, and thus absorb, the other person's pain and anxiety. If this happens, we lose our focus and cease to be a pure instrument for the universal healing force. I will keep returning to this issue throughout the following chapters, because learning Therapeutic Touch involves developing and reconciling these two qualities within ourselves.

The practitioner must also have a sense of confidence in the efficacy of Therapeutic Touch, that is, confidence in the existence of the universal life energy, in the intrinsic healing potential of all living things, and in his own ability to be an instrument of healing. Without such confidence or inner certainty it would be impossible to establish a clear intent to direct the energy for a therapeutic purpose. This confidence, however, must be based not on blind belief but on knowledge and experience. I will teach you what I know to be true from my own practice and at first you may have to give me the benefit of the doubt. But if the process is to be at all meaningful, you must, in the end, apply it in your own life and validate it for yourself.

3

The Method

Remember that there is a universal power, a force that has order as its basis. To heal one must become attuned to that universal power.

DORA KUNZ

Within the context of Therapeutic Touch, "healing" means helping the patient to re-establish an open, balanced energy flow. To do this, we

- assess the quality of the person's energies, searching for areas of congestion, disorder, and deficit;
- clear away congestion;
- transfer the life energy into depleted areas;
- balance the energy flow.

These aspects of the method are not separate, sequential stages; they are interrelated processes that are often performed simultaneously, in one coordinated gesture. For the purpose of teaching, however, I will discuss each aspect individually so that you will clearly understand its nature and purpose. With practice, you will gradually see for yourself how all these processes reinforce each other, forming an intricate and ordered interplay.

This book is not, by any means, a definitive text to be copied or mastered at once. Think of the detailed descriptions as a reference or resource to help you as your potential gradually unfolds. As is the case with dancing, swimming, or riding a bicycle, you learn Therapeutic Touch by getting the "feel" of it. You should not become discouraged, therefore, if you do not appreciate all the subtle nuances in the beginning, but simply go ahead and treat whatever area calls forth a response. I would urge you to practice regularly, for with Therapeutic Touch, as with any art form, one's ability grows in proportion to one's dedication and experience.

Preparing for the Treatment

The first requisite when practicing Therapeutic Touch is a calm, focused state of being. Remember that our thoughts and emotions are not confined within us but overflow into the atmosphere, so to speak, and influence others who are near us. If we are upset, anxious, or in a negative frame of mind, we will affect the patient adversely: the disturbances in our energy field will tend to amplify the disturbances within the patient's field.

The best preparation for the treatment, therefore, is to perform a short focusing or centering exercise— *especially if you are feeling upset or anxious in any way.* One helpful exercise, which has been used for years in the Therapeutic Touch workshops, is the following:

1) Sit comfortably and close your eyes.
2) Inhale and exhale deeply; and then
3) Focus your mind on some image in nature, such as a tree or a mountain, which brings you a sense of peace. If you become distracted, gently bring your mind back to your image of peace. Remember not to tighten up or try to force your mind to be still. Just maintain a calm but firm intent to keep focused on the image.

This technique will help you to quiet your mind and emotions, and also relax you physically. The amount of time spent on the exercise does not matter; it could last a few seconds or several minutes. What is important is that you feel a sense of peace and integrity, or wholeness, within yourself. It is this state of being that we call "centered." Because we are human beings, we will always be dealing with problems. However, if we can learn to quiet ourselves and feel a sense of inner peace and strength—that is, become centered—our personal anxieties will cease to dominate the foreground of our awareness. They will be relegated to the periphery of our minds and thus will not block or distort the healing energy as it flows through us.

If you feel that your patient needs some preparation for Therapeutic Touch, you could gently massage her neck and shoulders. Most people hold a great deal of tension in this area and if this is loosened, they will become more relaxed and will respond more quickly to the treatment. This brief massage also gives you the opportunity to make contact with the person and establish a spirit of mutual harmony; thus it will make you, also, more relaxed and less self-conscious. I cannot overemphasize the importance of this quality of inner rapport between practitioner and patient. If the energy transfer is to take place without disruption, we must "tune" ourselves, so to speak, to the rhythm of the patient. This does *not* mean focusing on the illness; on the contrary, it means acknowledging the true individuality or essence of the other person—which is much deeper and more inclusive than the illness. For it is this creative core of wholeness, this inner tendency toward order that we must try to strengthen through the healing process.

Assessing

The life energy, which flows through and extends beyond the patient's physical body, is felt most easily when the hands are held about three to five inches from the surface of the skin. If the hands are held closer, the texture of clothes and the sensation of body heat will be distracting; farther away, the energy is more diffuse and thus less easily perceived. Even when the patient's ailment is known to reside in a certain area of the body (such as a headache), the person's *entire* field must be assessed. Since the energy system is a dynamic, interconnected pattern, our concern is with the balance of the whole.

The Gesture

The physical movements of the assessment are very simple. In the beginning they may feel somewhat awkward, but after you have practiced for a short time, they will become very natural, and you will not be self-

conscious about them. The assessment can be made in one of two ways:
(see Diagram A)

1) Ask the patient to sit on a stool or sideways on a chair so that his back is unobstructed.
2) Sit or kneel to the side of the patient so that one of your hands — either the right or the left — extends in front of the patient and the other is behind his back.
3) Pass your hands gently through the patient's energy field (about three to five inches from the surface of the skin), palms facing his body, starting from the top of the head and moving down to the feet; when the hand in back reaches the patient's hips, keep it there while the other hand passes all the way down the legs to the feet.

or

(see Diagram B)

1) Ask the patient to sit on a stool or sideways on a chair.
2) Sit or kneel in front of the patient; pass your hands, parallel to each other with palms facing the patient, through the patient's energy field from head to foot; and then
3) Go in back of the patient and pass your hands, in the same manner, from the patient's head down to the hips.

Each of these approaches has a certain advantage. With the first, the cues (the characteristics described in the next section) are more easily perceived. When our

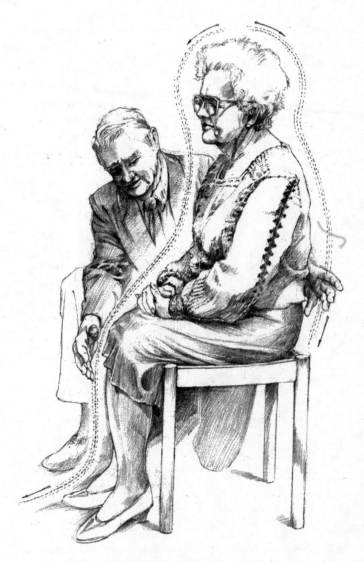

Diagram A: Assessing the Patient's Field with Hands
Opposite Each Other

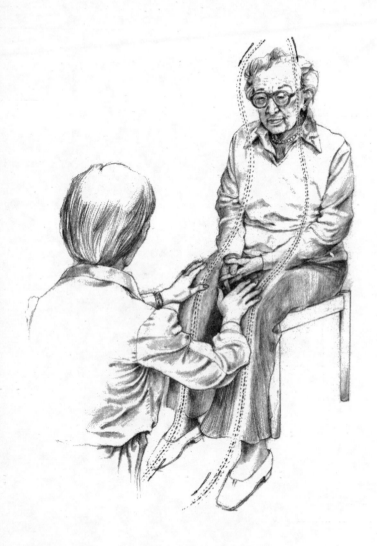

Diagram B: Assessing the Patient's Field with Hands
                    Parallel to Each Other

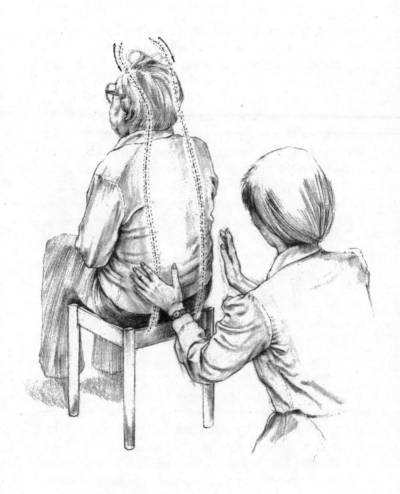

two hands are opposite each other they have a polar effect, intensifying the flow of energy between them and making the cues more palpable. However, with the second approach, since our two hands are side by side, we can better sense any differences between the right and left sides of the patient. (One way to gain both these advantages is to work with another practitioner. Since team-treating can be very effective, it will be be discussed in some depth in the next chapter.) A bedridden patient who cannot sit up can be asked to turn onto one side, so that it is possible to assess with one hand in front and one hand in back. When assessing and treating bedridden patients, make sure your own posture is comfortable. Otherwise you may not only be distracted by your discomfort but you may also constrict the energy flow.

Assessing should be done fairly quickly, in no more than fifteen to twenty seconds. If you move too slowly, you can easily lose your spontaneity and become self-conscious. On the other hand, if you move too quickly, you may race past the cues without picking them up. When assessing, it is important to move your hands in a smooth, light, downward motion. If your gestures are awkward and/or choppy, they will tend to irritate patients, for even when assessing you are still interacting with the patient's field and thus changing, to some extent, the pattern of the energy flow. Because the cues are very subtle, many beginners, in their effort to pick them up, bear down much too heavily or intensely. This can, unfortunately, give the patient an uncomfortable feeling of pressure or a sense of being closed in upon, especially if his energy field is congested. As will be described later, the energy congestion is carried out of the patient by bringing it down through the extremities. If you make a habit of moving your hands downward while assessing, any loose congestion that is dislodged will tend to go in the proper direction. If you move your hands around in circles or up and down while assessing, they may only stir up the congestion, thereby making the patient even more uncomfortable. Remember that the life energy is a continuum, and thus whatever we do to the patient's field around the body will have a definite physical effect. This may surprise you at first, but after you practice for a while you will begin to understand through experience that there is really no boundary between "inside" and "outside" but only one continuous energy flow—that is, the field.

The Cues

When you assess a really healthy person, you will feel the energy flowing in a balanced manner, which is evidenced either as a soft warmth or as a gentle vibration. In my classes I have noticed that students seem to feel the flow in either one or the other of these ways, but not in both. A healthy energy flow feels unbroken, evenly distributed, and comfortable in your hands. It also feels expansive because the exchange between the individual and the environment is open and free. When you assess people who are ill, you will pick up a number of different sensations, or cues, which indicate problems with the energy flow. These cues are qualitative and therefore difficult to describe precisely in single words; because of this, I will often use several words to help clarify the description. To make it easier for you to distinguish among them, I have divided the cues into four broad categories: loose congestion, tight congestion, deficit, and imbalance. In actual practice, however, these cues are not separate but tend to merge into one another.

LOOSE CONGESTION: This feels something like a cloud or a wave of heat, thickness, pressure, or heaviness. If a person has a wound or an infection, loose congestion can often be found around its area. However, it can also be "free-floating"—that is, found over areas where there is no known physical problem. The quality of the congestion varies from patient to patient; for example, with some patients it may be felt as heat and with others as thickness. It is also possible for two practitioners to feel the same patient's condition differently: one might sense it as heaviness and another as pressure. The reason for this may be that people tend to interpret and describe sensations in different ways. In any case, no matter how one senses and describes the loose congestion, its treatment is always the same.

TIGHT CONGESTION: If the congestion settles or becomes lodged in a specific area, it blocks the flow of the life energy. Therefore, if you feel the baseline flow as warm, the blocked area will feel cold; if you feel the energy flow as a rhythmic vibration, the blocked area will give you no response or seem to be a void. Individuals with chronic problems generally suffer from these energy blockages; if you assessed someone with ulcerative colitis, for example, you would most probably feel a sense of coldness or emptiness around the intestinal area. Often there is not a sharp division between a flowing area and a blocked area. Thus when assessing the energy field of a person with pneumonia, you may feel a coldness over the affected part of the lung, indicating a blockage due to infection, and also a coolness over the surrounding areas, indicating a sluggishness of flow. It really does not matter, however, whether or not the Therapeutic Touch practitioner knows the person's medical diagnosis, such as "left lower lobe pneumonia." What is important is that she find the energy blockages and try to clear them so that a balanced flow can be restored. Sometimes, on initial assessment, a cloud of loose congestion lies on top of some blocked congestion; the coldness is thus not perceptible until the thickness, heat, or pressure has been cleared away. This illustrates the point mentioned earlier: that one must assess continually — not just once at the beginning of the treatment.

DEFICIT: Illness is always associated with a depletion of vital energy. The deficit is most easily perceived around a problem area, such as the site of a wound or infection, but of course a deficit in one place debilitates the whole person. On assessment, a deficit can be felt as a drawing or pulling sensation, as though a stream of very fine water bubbles were being pulled through one's hands. Sometimes the hands seem to be magnetically drawn to a particular part of the patient's body. On other occasions the deficit may be felt as a hollowness; this is quite different from the lack of response of a blocked area, for it produces a distinct impression that the area is open and actively pulling in the energy. Deficits, however, are almost always found *underneath* heavily congested or blocked areas. Remember that health is associated with a constant energy interchange with the environment.

Congestion interferes with this interchange, thus creating a deficit of energy within the individual. When loose or blocked congestion is released during a treatment, the area opens up and you may then feel a pulling or drawing sensation caused by the underlying deficit. If an area is partially blocked, the initial assessment will sometimes produce both the pulling of the deficit and the coldness of the resistance created by the tight congestion.

IMBALANCE: The fourth type of cue or sensation you may pick up is imbalance, caused when a particular area in the energy field is not flowing in harmony with the whole. One frequently finds this around the area of a malfunctioning organ. A common type of imbalance produces an area of static or pins and needles, which is prickly and uncomfortable to one's hands. In another type of imbalance, the energy seems to flap or surge in and out in a disorganized manner. It is important to remember that the cues are not sharply delineated; they tend to overlap and blur into one another. For example, you might feel an area of thickness, indicating loose congestion, which is interspersed or overlaid with the pins and needles of disorder. I have sometimes felt a filmy type of agitation in the field, which could be labeled as either congestion, imbalance, or both. Thus one could say in general that when you pick up an area that gives you any distinct abnormal sensation, this is an area that needs attention since, broadly speaking, any type of problem puts the system out of balance. Energies should flow in an even, orderly manner; even if only one area is blocked, the system as a whole is not in balance. The entire Therapeutic Touch process, therefore, is an attempt to re-establish dynamic balance within the field.

Validating the Assessment

Your assessment of the quality of the patient's energy flow can be validated in several ways, each of which has certain advantages and disadvantages. For example, since the treatment is based on the assessment, if your patient responds and feels better, your assessment was probably correct. However, as mentioned before, the patient may not respond very well even when the assessment is very good and the treatment beautifully given. It is also possible for the patient to be helped quite a bit from a treatment based on a superficial assessment. It seems that a patient's intrinsic tendency toward wholeness (his inner wisdom) can compensate to a remarkable degree for our lack of assessment and treatment skills. This is an important point, which should reassure all practitioners—beginners and experienced alike.

As the energy field perspective does not exactly match the medical perspective, one has to be careful about trying to validate a Therapeutic Touch assessment by comparing it with the patient's medical diagnosis. It is true that there are direct correspondences between the two because if an organ is malfunctioning, there is generally a problem with the energy flow in that particular area. (Hepatitis, for example, is associated with an imbalanced, sluggish energy flow in and around the liver.) Sometimes, however, the energy assessment will differ from the medical diagnosis. I once treated a young woman diagnosed as having strep throat. She had completed a full course of antibiotics, but her throat was still sore and she felt very tired. When assessing her energy field, I could find no problem in the area of her throat.

However, her chest, stomach, and intestines were quite thick and heavy, which indicated loose congestion in these areas; her kidneys were cold, which indicated a blockage, and her legs and feet were sluggish and cool. In this case, the diagnosis of strep throat was not helpful in validating the Therapeutic Touch assessment because the main energy problem was the tight congestion in the kidney area, which was blocking the energy flow. When this was loosened and the congestion cleared from the young woman's field, her sore throat improved very quickly. In this situation, therefore, my assessment was validated by the results of the treatment.

This case points up the fact that the energy assessment does not always correspond to the patient's symptoms. This young woman did not feel anything in her kidneys; she was aware of a sore throat, some chest congestion, and general fatigue. In other instances, however, the pattern of the energy flow corresponds very well with the patient's symptoms. One man, for example, came for treatment because of a pain in the area of his right kidney for which no medical diagnosis could be made. On assessment, I felt a nothingness or emptiness in that particular area, which indicated a blockage of the energy flow. When this blockage was loosened and the energy started to flow actively again, the man experienced relief from pain. Thus my assessment was validated both by the patient's symptoms and by the results of the treatment. Cases such as this suggest that there can be imbalances in the flow of the life energy, which, although creating discomfort for the patient, are not associated with enough physical damage to be picked up on a medical diagnostic test.

You can also compare your impressions with those

of another Therapeutic Touch practitioner. This is a helpful means of validation because you and your partner are both looking at the patient from the same perspective. When two experienced practitioners assess a patient, there is usually very little discrepancy between the two impressions; different words may be used but the underlying meaning is the same. In a beginners' workshop, however, there may be discrepancies when two students assess the same patient. The students generally find the correct area but may interpret the signals differently. Some students are initially more sensitive to certain cues than to others; it takes some practice for them to round out their sensitivity so that they read all the cues with equal skill. It is often the case that congestion, deficit, and disorder can be found in the same area of the ill person's energy field, so it is not surprising that beginners' assessments show some discrepancies. We must also recognize the fact that we know, on an inner level, much more than we can describe verbally. I have found from my own practice that the best Therapeutic Touch treatments are given when the conscious, rational mind is in harmony with the silent voice of the intuition, and the hands are effortlessly guided from within.

Assessing with Your Whole Being

The first requisite in assessment is a quiet, listening attitude. The cues are subtle, and we will not be able to pick them up if our thoughts are scattered and noisy. When we listen to music, we hear the pattern of sound waves with our ears, but we also experience the quality of the composition on many different levels. Similarly, when we assess the patient's energy flow, we pick up certain cues with our hands, but we also experience a range of nuances which are integrated into a whole. When we are near people, our continually interacting energies make it possible for us to feel their love and joy as well as their anxiety and depression, even though no words have been exchanged. This is especially true during Therapeutic Touch because of the intensity of the interaction between the patient and practitioner. If the patient is very anxious, you may feel it as a sensation of static in your hands or it may reach you as a general impression.

As you listen, so to speak, to the melody of the patient's energy field, you may see images spontaneously appearing in your mind's eye. These internal images, like the external cues, can give you valuable information about the person you are treating. One student said that he saw streams of white light flowing through the patient's entire body except for the upper right abdominal area, which was grey and static. In this case the inner visualization corresponded to the patient's physical condition, which was a mild case of hepatitis. Sometimes an image may convey a person's general character. Once, while assessing a patient, I saw a beautiful flower in full bloom; it was not a real flower, however, but was made of porcelain. This suggested to me that the patient, although blossoming in the prime of life, was actually quite delicate and fragile. Since this image was consistent with some other information I had about the patient, I was extremely gentle with the treatment. Such images, like all other cues, must be personally interpreted and validated by the practitioner whenever possible. Many are associative, arising from our own daily experiences and interests, and some may even mislead us if we take them too seriously. Thus, like everything connected with an undertaking as subjective as Therapeutic Touch, images and symbols must be evaluated within the context of the treatment situation as a whole.

Practice Exercise

At this point, you have enough information to begin assessing people for yourself. Remember to perform your preparatory exercise, because assessing is dependent on a relaxed body and a calm, open mind. The process also requires spontaneity. We have found that the best initial assessments are done by passing the hands through the patient's field *once;* if you go over the patient again and again you will tend to become stale and self-conscious. The initial assessment should give you enough information to begin the treatment, during which the energy flow will change and thus require further assessment. Assessing is always an ongoing process, so you need not be anxious about picking up all the cues at once.

When you start assessing, you may find that one of your hands is more sensitive than the other, as sometimes happens when people begin learning Therapeutic Touch. After a little practice, however, both hands become equally sensitive to the cues. You may also become aware of a gentle tingling sensation in your hands, which is the feeling of your own energy flow. During assessment, this sensation serves as a baseline; your energies interpenetrate those of the patient and whatever feels different from your own emanation is a characteristic of the other person.

If you find that, in becoming receptive to the patient's condition, you start to absorb the problem (for instance, you become upset, tired, and/or develop an ache or a pain somewhere), stop assessing immediately, take a deep breath, and re-center yourself. Remember that you must not only be sensitive and empathetic, but also focused and integrated.

The chart on the next page may be helpful as a review and point of reference.

Clearing Loose Congestion

When passing your hands through a person's energy field, you may feel waves or clouds of thickness, heaviness, pressure, or heat in certain areas. These cues indicate the loose congestion mentioned earlier. It is not the same as physical congestion; however, since the life energy penetrates and interacts with the physical body, wherever there is physical congestion there is usually energy congestion as well. Energy congestion, on the whole, is more generalized throughout the body than its physical counterpart; thus, if someone has a stuffy nose you may find heat or thickness all around the head, not simply over the nose. Sometimes there is a degree of energy congestion that does not seem to have a physical counterpart. The patients are often aware of the condition, however, because when it is removed many report that they feel lighter and more expansive.

Energy congestion tends to travel from the head downward. It is easily cleared from the person's field with repeated gentle, sweeping, downward motions of the hands. If you feel that the substance is sticking to

How to Recognize a Patient's Cues

TYPE OF IMBALANCE	CUE *(may be experienced as ...)*
Loose congestion	Heat Thickness Heaviness Pressure
Tight congestion or obstruction	Coldness Blankness No movement Emptiness
Partially obstructed or sluggish area	Coolness Decrease in intensity of energy rhythm
Deficit	Open hole Pulling or drawing
Local imbalance	Pins and needles Static Break in rhythm Mixed-up or disordered vibrations

your hands, simply shake it off at the end of each stroke or whenever it seems to have accumulated, just as you shake off water when your hands are wet. Think of the congestion as leaving the patient and dissipating into the environment. Do not let it become lodged in your hands because, besides creating discomfort, it may dull your sensitivity and block the energy flow. I find that although some of the congestion travels down the person's arms and out the hands, most of it goes through the trunk, down the legs, and out the feet. It is important to remove it *completely* from the person—not just push it from one place to another. I have sometimes seen beginning students clear the patient's lung area of congestion only to make the person nauseated by allowing it to settle around the area of the stomach. If the person has head or chest congestion, you can take it out sideways to avoid the discomfort of moving it all down through the stomach. When you do this, however, you will find that some of it invariably escapes downward and must be cleared through the legs and feet.

If the person's feet are blocked (that is, if they feel blank or cold), the loose congestion cannot be completely removed until the blockage is released. It is best to remove a foot blockage as soon as possible, because if you bring more congestion down into the area, the patient may experience an uncomfortable sensation of pressure building up in his legs and feet. A foot blockage is generally released by exerting a gentle pressure with one's fingers under the arches of the patient's feet (see Diagram C). By holding this area steadily, you will stimulate the energy flow and the feet should warm up in a short time. If you are trained in massage therapy, you can gently massage the feet; this will facilitate the release

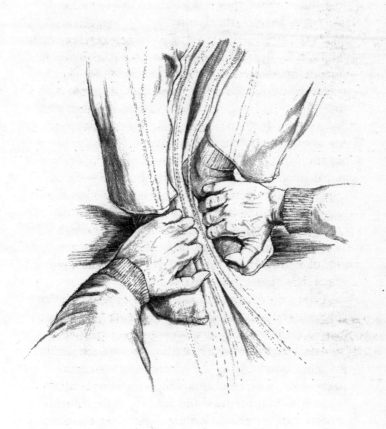

Diagram C: Enhancing the Energy Flow at the Feet

of the tight congestion and allow the energy to flow more freely. It is a good practice to check the energy flow in both legs carefully, because sometimes another area (often around the ankles) is blocked and needs to be loosened as described above.

You can also visualize the energy flowing freely through the legs and feet, as a stream of light or a current of water. Images such as these are dynamic energy patterns, which, if formed and projected with a specific intent, can help to guide the energy flow within the patient's field. When using imagery, however, it is essential that you visualize the result that you are trying to achieve, that is, the resolution of the energy problem and the balancing of the patient's field. If you concentrate on the problem and think of the person as ill, two things will tend to happen: (1) your effort will become fragmented because your thinking is contrary to your general intent to re-establish wholeness, and (2) your negative thought pattern will reinforce the patient's imbalance. Thus, once again, learning to become an instrument of healing involves learning to consciously control our thoughts and to use them for a therapeutic purpose.

Most patients with tension headaches have a buildup of tight congestion in the shoulders and/or the feet. Because of these blockages, the loose congestion tends to back up into the head instead of moving downward. When treating a person with a tension headache, I massage the neck and shoulders, unblock the feet, and remove the loose congestion from the entire energy field. When clearing the head area, our gestures should be very gentle and rhythmical. It is best to work fairly quickly and remove our hands from the area as soon as the pressure has been relieved. The head is very sensitive, and if we work there too long the patient may become groggy and/or irritable. The person will often sense a release of congestion and will report that the headache is draining. Children, in particular, are sensitive to the energy flow and will often give very helpful feedback. I will never forget the little girl who exclaimed, in the middle of a treatment, "Now my headache is in my knees!" I put my hands over her knees and, sure enough, felt a sensation of heat. When this was cleared away, the headache (or kneeache) was completely gone.

Practice Exercise

People with the common cold generally have quite a lot of loose congestion in their energy fields. Therefore, I recommend calling up a friend who has a cold and asking if you can practice together. (Staying at home with a cold is very boring, so your friend may welcome an interesting diversion.) The following steps can be used as guidelines.

1) Perform your preliminary centering exercise. If you feel that your friend would be willing, you could both do it together.
2) Establish the intent to be an instrument of healing and to cooperate with Nature's tendency toward order and wholeness.
3) Gently massage her neck and shoulders.
4) When your friend seems more relaxed, assess the condition of her energy field.
5) Clear the field of any loose congestion.
6) Release any congestion that has collected in the feet.

7) Ask her for feedback.
8) Repeat any of the above steps as necessary.

As you remove the loose congestion, the pattern of the energy flow may change in unexpected ways. For example, the feet may be fairly warm at the beginning of the treatment, but as you bring down the congestion, it may become lodged in the feet and make them cold. As you work, therefore, you have to assess these changes and modify your treatment accordingly. (Although I have numbered the procedures in order to help you get started, you will soon realize that, in actual practice, they are not always performed in a sequential manner.) When the feet are unblocked and all the congestion is cleared away, the energy field becomes smoother and more rhythmical — and at this point you should stop.

If, during the process, you inadvertently absorb some of the congestion (for example, if your hand starts to hurt or if you get a headache, upset stomach, chest tightness, and so on), stop clearing the patient's field and clear your own instead! In such a case, take a deep breath and re-center yourself as I described earlier. You can also visualize the healing energy as a waterfall flowing from the top of your head down through your feet, washing all the congestion away. If you feel that your feet are blocked, you can visualize yourself as a tree with roots going deep into the ground; this will help open the energy flow at your feet so the congestion can drain.

Before you proceed to the next section, it would be helpful for you to clear the energy fields of several people who have headaches and colds. With a little practice, you will be less self-conscious about giving a treatment and more sensitive to the flow of the vital energy.

Transferring Energy

When people are ill, they are not adequately absorbing and processing the vital energy. Illness is therefore always associated with energy depletion. During a treatment we try to make the vital energy more accessible to the patient by consciously serving as an energy conductor and transformer. When transferring energy, it is essential that we establish the intent to become a conduit for a universal force. If we forget to do this, we will give our own energy to the patient and then feel tired and irritable after the treatment. Many practitioners find it helpful to visualize the energy as a stream of light coming from above, flowing through them and going into the patient. In any case, whether you use imagery or not, the intent to be a conductor is of the utmost importance. Since the energy first has to flow through our own field, we must try to stay calm and focused during the transfer. If we are anxious and constricted, we will block the energy; if we are distracted or in a state of inner conflict we will dissipate it. The flow of water through a pipe can be used as a simple metaphor. The pipe must be open, sound, and whole; if it is obstructed or leaky, the water will not reach the tap where it is needed. When we are relaxed and working in an integrated manner, the healing energy flows through us effortlessly and we, as well as the patients, are replenished.

Assessing the Deficits

The intent to be an energy conductor should be established at the very beginning of the treatment, even before the assessment is made. As soon as you move toward a person with a desire to help, he may unconsciously start drawing energy from you because compassion opens us up to one another. Therefore the transfer can start instantaneously and continue during the whole treatment, even though you may not be aware of it during the initial stages of assessment.

Since an individual's energy flow is an interconnected system, it is always the *whole* that is depleted of energy. However, in certain places there are openings, so to speak, into which the energy can be transferred most directly and effectively. Practitioners refer to these openings as depleted areas or deficits. An energy deficit is usually felt as a drawing or pulling sensation in a certain area of the field; however, your mind's eye might present an image that suggests a need for energy in some area or your intuition may simply guide your hand to a particular place. Deficits are often found around areas of wounds, infections, and malfunctioning organs. If there is loose congestion in the patient's field, first clear this away and then you will more easily feel the pulling sensation. It is important to assess the entire field for deficits because they can often be found in several areas at once. A person with asthma, for example, often needs energy in the areas around the stomach and kidneys as well as around the lungs.

Filling the Deficits

When you sense a pulling somewhere, leave your hand over that place so the patient can draw the energy through you (see Diagram D). Flowing movement of energy often feels like warm water bubbles going through your hands into the patient. Do not try to force it. If you remain

48

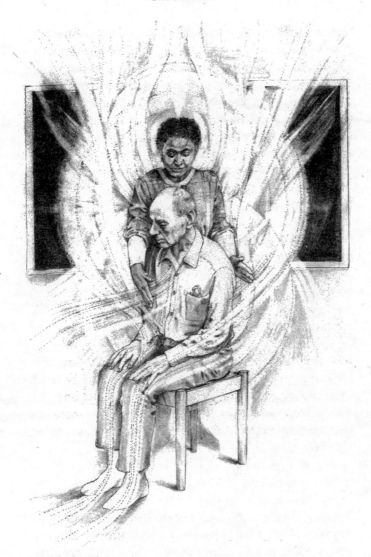

Diagram D: An Artist's Representation of the Energy
Transfer

relaxed and focused, the energy will flow naturally; if you push or strain you will constrict the flow and thus defeat your purpose. Remember that the patient is not passive or inert, but rather an active participant in the healing process. The patient pulls in the energy according to her condition at the moment: sometimes the flow is slow, sometimes fast; sometimes it moves continuously, sometimes in spurts; sometimes the bubbles are very fine and sometimes coarse. After a little while the flow will stop and the area will feel as though it has been filled in. At this point, you should reassess to see if there are other areas of depletion, in which case they should also be treated. Eventually, the pulling or drawing will stop, which indicates that the patient has absorbed all the energy she can assimilate at the moment.

The Acceleration of
the Healing Process

As discussed earlier, one essential characteristic of living organisms (that is, self-organizing wholes) is self-restoration or healing. When you send life energy into the patient, you help to strengthen the individual's intrinsic healing ability. Changes will therefore begin to take place spontaneously within the field. For example, more congestion generally surfaces and starts draining downward. It is helpful, at this point, to stop sending energy for a moment, clear the field, and then go back and resume filling in the deficit. Sometimes the congestion, moving downward, gets caught somewhere; this often happens in places where there is muscle tension, such as the area around the shoulder blades. The patient will feel this "caught" congestion as a sudden pain or pressure.

If this occurs, simply rub the area with your hands to loosen the congestion and then clear it out of the field. Because of these spontaneous changes, it is helpful to reassess the patient's entire field frequently during the treatment. One common mistake among beginners is to become completely engrossed in sending energy to an affected area and to forget about the balance of the whole. Remember, in particular, to check the energy flow at the patient's feet. If congestion drains downward and clogs in the feet, turning them cold, the person can become overloaded very quickly during an energy transfer.

Subjective Experiences of Patients

Many people say that they feel sensations of tingling and/or warmth when receiving the vital energy, and some also say that they can feel the loose congestion traveling down through their bodies. Most people relax during a Therapeutic Touch treatment—especially when the energy starts flowing into them—and many will report typical sensations of relaxation: their hands and feet become warm and heavy, their breathing becomes deeper, their stomachs rumble, and so on. Sometimes patients release tension in little spurts and may experience some muscle twitching or shivering. Most people are not bothered by these sensations, but if you are treating someone who is not familiar with techniques which induce a relaxation response, you may want to reassure him that these are common experiences. You need not be concerned, however, if your patient has no particular sensation. The treatment works whether the patient feels anything or not.

Regulating the Amount of Energy

Healing energy, like air, water, and food, is an essential form of nourishment which must be correctly regulated. Taking in too much energy, like eating too much, is not only uncomfortable but also unhealthy. There appears to be an unconscious regulatory process, an energy appetite, so to speak, which controls the intake of the life force. Therefore, most of the time the pulling sensation automatically stops when the patient has taken in as much as can be assimilated. At this point the patient will often say that he feels full, or has had enough. As is the case with food, a certain amount of energy is necessary to digest and assimilate the new input. Because of this, you will find that very debilitated persons can process only a small amount of energy at any one time, even though they apparently need a great deal. It is best to give such people short, gentle treatments at frequent intervals.

It is very important to be sensitive to the tapering off and cessation of the energy pull. If you disregard this and try to force more into the patient, he may become restless, irritable, and then dizzy or lightheaded. Some people are very sensitive and a sudden large input of energy can overwhelm their regulatory processes; thus they can become overloaded *while* they are still drawing energy through you. It is a good idea, therefore, to check periodically how the person is feeling, and if he is becoming overloaded, stop and have him sit quietly in a comfortable chair or lie down. We have found that "energy indigestion" only lasts for a short time (generally a few minutes), but as this experience can be upsetting, it is important that you explain what has happened and offer support and reassurance.

Loosening Tight Congestion

You will frequently come upon a feeling of coldness or blankness over certain areas, which indicates that the energy flow is obstructed. In order to assist the healing process, we must try to loosen these areas because they are impeding the proper circulation of the energy and the drainage of congestion. A blockage is released by physically loosening the area, in various ways, which I will describe, and/or by sending the life energy directly into it. Just as a stream of water can penetrate and loosen hard, impacted earth, so can a stream of the life energy penetrate and loosen the tightness. When sending the energy, however, you must think of it going *deeply* into the affected area. No matter how solid the obstruction appears to be, the life energy — following your intent — can go into it.

You have already experienced releasing a tight area when you massaged your patient's shoulders. An accumulation of muscle tension obstructs the circulation of blood and lymph, as well as the circulation of the vital energy. When you rubbed the shoulder area, you loosened both the physical and vital congestion and therefore improved the energy flow. Also, when the blockage was loosened, congestion that was trapped in the patient's head could proceed to drain. This is why many people report that their clogged heads and headaches are relieved when their shoulders are massaged.

An area that often becomes tightly congested is the solar plexus (the stomach/intestinal area). We all know that when we get nervous we tend to tighten up in the middle and feel "butterflies" in our stomachs.[20] Prolonged tension held in this area can lead to digestive disorders and to other serious problems such as ulcers and colitis. Since any kind of illness is upsetting and stressful, I find that patients in general tend to have a sluggish energy flow in the solar plexus. To loosen this area, put one hand in front — directly over the cool or blank spot — and put the other hand in back to support the patient. (In my own practice, I generally touch the patient physically when doing this.) Then attune to the universal source and direct a stream of energy into the tightness. Remember that the energy will follow your intent. If you want to use additional imagery, you can visualize light shining through darkness, a knot unraveling, a logjam breaking up in a river, or, better yet, any appropriate image that spontaneously appears in your mind's eye. As the vital energy penetrates the tightness, several processes are simultaneously set in motion: (a) the impacted congestion becomes looser, that is, it becomes hot and thick in your hands, and you must bring it down and out through the patient's feet; (b) as the area opens up, you will feel a pull as the person begins actively to draw energy through you; (c) the patient will start to show some of the signs of relaxation, which I mentioned earlier. After a little while the pull will diminish, the congestion will lessen, and then you will know that it is time to stop. As many people hold emotional tension in the solar plexus, this is generally a very vulnerable area; therefore, when working in this region, be as gentle and supportive as possible.

When someone is ill, the kidney area is frequently blocked. This is especially true after surgery, after taking antibiotics, and if the patient has had an infection, particularly in the kidneys. To loosen the congestion, I find it helpful to rub the kidney area of the back physically with either a circular or an up-down motion. When the area feels a little warmer, I visualize the healing energy streaming through it. As the congestion is loosened, heat is generally felt at the person's back; however, it can also come out in front and start moving down the legs. For this reason, remember to keep reassessing the field—both in front and in back—at regular intervals, and releasing the energy via the feet.

If a person has a chronic lung disease such as emphysema or cystic fibrosis, or even an acute problem such as pneumonia or bronchitis, the lung area will feel cold and without movement, indicating an obstruction of both the physical and vital circulation. In such cases a gentle, rhythmical percussion or tapping on the patient's chest will loosen the congestion, often causing him to cough. When the chest area is clearer, the person can actively pull in the life energy. You can facilitate the energy transfer by visualizing the lungs filled with the life energy and functioning in a healthy manner.

When the life energy begins to penetrate a thickly congested or blocked area, the patient will often report a sensation of heat, which disappears when the congestion is finally loosened. People are generally not bothered by this experience, but if the heat intensifies into an uncomfortable burning sensation, it is helpful to visualize the vital energy as a dark but vivid blue, such as one sees in stained-glass windows. Every color has a specific frequency, and it has been found that the frequency corresponding to a cobalt or sapphire blue has a very cooling and soothing effect. Sometimes the patient may report discomfort when energy is transferred into an infected wound or abscess. If visualizing blue light does not relieve the discomfort, direct the energy into another receptive place such as the kidneys. As mentioned before in the case of infection, the kidney/adrenal area tends to draw a great deal of energy. Remember to keep in mind the fact that we are not treating the wound or the infection, but the entire organism; and if we help to strengthen the whole, the condition of the part will improve.

It is important to loosen a blocked area very early in the course of the treatment because it will impede both the transfer of energy and the drainage of the congestion. When you come upon a cold or blank area, do not tense up and try to force the energy in; paradoxically, the more you force the less will happen. Stay relaxed, make a clear intent to penetrate the area, and the universal energy will do the work through you. Sometimes the blockage is superficial and will release very quickly. As soon as you direct energy into the area, the tight congestion will turn into loose congestion (heat or thickness) and the energy flow will improve (the coldness will turn into warmth or the blankness will turn into a flowing vibration). At other times, however, the blockage may be deep, especially if the patient has a chronic disease. When this is the case, it will generally not loosen completely in one treatment; you will have to unravel it gradually with regular treatments over an extended period of time. If you find that the person is blocked in two places, it is generally best to loosen the lower one first because, if you initially loosen the upper one, the lower blockage will prevent the congestion from moving downward. If one area is open and actively pulls energy while another area is obstructed, I would release the tight area first; in this way any congestion that surfaces during the transfer can be cleared without difficulty.

Balancing the Field

There is often a feeling of pins and needles in some area of the energy field, which generally indicates a localized imbalance—a rough edge, so to speak. You can easily smooth this out with a gentle stroking motion of your hands. However, since any kind of problem puts the system out of balance, the whole treatment is essentially a rebalancing of the energy field. You unblock the obstructions, fill in the depleted areas, and smooth the rough edges until the entire field is flowing in an open, continuous manner. It is essential that you find the problem areas and work on them, but it should always be for the purpose of making the whole more integrated. For example, many people hold more tension on one side than another, so on assessment you will often find one side to be cooler than the other. Knowing that coolness indicates a sluggish energy flow, you can visualize the life energy streaming through the affected side until the temperature is equalized.

I have always found Therapeutic Touch to be an aesthetic as well as a scientific process, since its purpose is to create or re-establish harmony, balance, and proportion, all of which are attributes of the beautiful. In some ways, this method of healing is a form of dynamic sculpture. Just as the image of the whole statue always dominates the details in the sculptor's mind, so the image or idea of balanced wholeness is the practitioner's overriding concern. The difference is that the "statue," in our case, is a co-creator in the healing process, because the inner tendency toward order and balance exists within all living creatures, no matter how obstructed or fragmented they may appear to be. As with any creative process, our task is not to "do" the healing but to help it emerge from within the patient himself.

> It results from this that perfection of invention touches hands with absence of invention, as if that line which the human eye will follow with effortless delight were a line that had not been invented but simply discovered, had in the beginning been hidden by nature and in the end been found by the engineer. There is an ancient myth about the image asleep in the block of marble until it is carefully disengaged by the sculptor. The sculptor must himself feel that he is not so much inventing or shaping the curve of breast or shoulder as delivering the image from its prison.[21]

When a person's energies have become more balanced, it seems that his inner essence is, so to speak, delivered from its prison. Many patients are in fact surprised, as though they are discovering something new about themselves: an inner peace, buoyancy, and clarity, hitherto hidden within, can now come forth. And it is at this point that the most profound healing begins to occur, for from this deeper dimension of consciousness comes creative insight and the power to break through old habit patterns associated with disease. During Therapeutic Touch, therefore, we must try always to think of the individual as being synchronized on all levels: physical, psychological, and intuitional/ spiritual.

Ending the Treatment

"How long does it take to give a treatment?" "When should I stop?" These questions are raised by all beginning students. My colleagues and I have found that as every treatment is unique, each will unfold itself or run its course in its own particular amount of time. It is true that there are some general patterns: the average treatment for an adult is about fifteen to twenty minutes; children are smaller and generally more sensitive, so a little child might be balanced in about five minutes, and the treatment of a premature baby should only take a few seconds. People respond so differently, however, that it is inappropriate to try to determine the length of a treatment by the clock. Even if we had to rely on clock time it would be extremely difficult to do so because during Therapeutic Touch, time seems to disappear. We experience the stopping of time — the eternal moment — not just during Therapeutic Touch but whenever we are doing something that we thoroughly enjoy for its own sake. When the activity is over, we do not know whether one minute or twenty minutes has elapsed because time is irrelevant. If at some point during a treatment I start to become conscious of the passing of time, it invariably means that the patient's energies are almost in balance and that the treatment is drawing to a close.

Therefore when students ask "When should I stop?" the only answer I can give is, "Stop when you are finished." When the energy field is finally balanced, there is an unmistakable "finished" feeling, similar to an artist's perception of when his work is done. Such a feeling of resolution is also experienced after a meaningful conversation, when all has been said for the moment;

tomorrow, of course, there might be more to say, but for now we feel satisfied. In the same way, the patient may need another treatment tomorrow, but for now the healing is completed.

Sometimes, however, we have to stop the treatment before it has run its full course. This can happen if the tension release gets too intense (for example, if the amount of shivering or muscle twitching that the individual is experiencing is too uncomfortable) or if the person is very sensitive to a sudden input of energy and becomes overloaded. It can also happen that, even though the patient is not showing any signs of discomfort, our intuition will tell us to stop early. If ever you are in doubt as to whether to proceed, just stop; self-doubt leads to fragmentation, which diminishes the effectiveness of the treatment. If you stop before you feel that the person's energies are in balance, this does not necessarily mean that the treatment was not fulfilled. From one perspective it is true that the treatment did not follow a normal course, but from another perspective the treatment was right because you did what seemed best for the patient. Moreover, if you give the treatment wholeheartedly, you will feel an intrinsic satisfaction in the process itself; fulfillment, then, does not come *afterwards* but is experienced *during* the treatment, at every moment.

To help the new energy pattern establish itself within the field, it is important for patients to rest for about twenty to thirty minutes after the treatment. Most people actually feel like resting, just as if they had finished a heavy meal. Sometimes the effects of the treatment are not felt by the patient until the energy is somewhat assimilated. If, therefore, you feel the person's energy

field is balanced and yet she tells you that the headache is still there, do not continue the treatment against
your better judgment. If you ask the person to sit quietly,
the headache will probably disappear within a few
minutes. Remember that you do not have to do everything yourself. The healing momentum, which has been
quickened during Therapeutic Touch, will continue well
beyond the limited time of the treatment. The words of
Lao Tsu, the ancient sage, are very appropriate in this
connection:

> *Creating, yet not possessing,*
> *Working, yet not taking credit.*
> *Work is done, then forgotten.*
> *Therefore it lasts forever.*[22]

Summary

In the beginning, Therapeutic Touch may seem compli-
cated and difficult, but after you practice for a while you
will begin to realize its essential simplicity. For review,
I will quickly go through the treatment with you, so you
can get a better sense of how the process flows. Remember that the ability to heal is already there within you,
as a latent capacity, and you have only to bring it
forth.

- Perform your preliminary relaxation exercise and feel
  yourself to be a center of peace.
- Direct your intent toward becoming a vehicle for the
  universal life energy.
- Gently massage the patient's neck and shoulders.
- When the patient seems more relaxed, assess the quality of his energy system.

- Clear away any loose congestion (thickness, heat, pressure), making sure that the energy is flowing freely through the feet.
- Loosen any obstructions (cold or blank areas) so that the field is open and flowing.
- Fill in depleted areas, where you feel a pulling sensation, drawing from the universal field.
- If you become drained of your own energy or if you absorb the patient's problem, stop immediately and rebalance yourself.
- Reassess the patient's field from time to time and clear away any more congestion that has surfaced.
- Observe the patient for signs of relaxation (such as deeper breathing, face flushing, muscle twitching).
- Ask for feedback from the patient and modify the treatment accordingly.
- Think of the person as being well and balanced on all levels.
- Conclude the treatment when the deficits have been filled in and the energy system is flowing in a more open, even manner.
- Ask the patient to sit quietly or lie down for twenty to thirty minutes.

These steps, of course, are not always performed sequentially, and the more you practice, the more you will integrate them into one continuous, flowing movement.

4

Therapeutic Touch in Daily Practice

*The gift which is given without thought of recom-
pense, in the belief that it ought to be made, in a fit
place, at an opportune time and to a deserving
person—such a gift is Pure.*

BHAGAVAD GITA

Once you start to practice Therapeutic Touch on a
regular basis, certain practical issues may arise. The
material in this chapter has come from my own experience as a practitioner and from discussions with colleagues and students. Since Therapeutic Touch is based
on a universal human interaction, practitioners tend to
experience the same problems, voice the same concerns,
and ask the same questions.

For example, in almost every class someone asks,
"What is the best way to explain Therapeutic Touch to a
friend or patient?" There are many good ways of doing
this and, since people are so different, our explanations
should always suit the individual occasion. Once, when
I was a beginner, I wanted to help a little boy with a
stomach ache. It was the first time I had introduced

Therapeutic Touch to a child, so I was a little uncertain. "Can I put my hand on the place where you hurt?" I asked. He nodded his head, so I put my hand on his stomach. Then, not knowing what his response would be, I lifted my hand a few inches from the surface of his body and said, "You know, I can feel your pain all the way out here." He nodded his head again, looking at me as if I had just made the most obvious statement in the world! After I recovered from my initial surprise, I relaxed completely and gave him a good treatment. I realized later on that the little boy had taught me a lesson: Therapeutic Touch is a normal, natural process and if I could convey a simple, matter-of-fact attitude about it, just as he did, this would affect people more deeply than my words.

This does not mean, however, that words are unimportant. On the contrary, I feel we have to be very careful about what we say to patients. I have found that, initially, a fairly simple explanation is best. You might say something to the effect that Therapeutic Touch is a method of balancing life energy, which many nurses are now using in their work. You could then wait and see how the person responds. Some people want to know a great many details while others only want you to help them feel better. You can also say, quite honestly, that you have just read this book and would appreciate the opportunity to practice. If the person knows that you are a beginner, he will not expect a spectacular result. This can be helpful because if you know that someone has a high expectation you may tend to worry too much about fulfilling it. It is essential not to make any definite claims, but rather to try to convey the idea that Therapeutic Touch is an open-ended, joint endeavor. "Let's try it together and see what happens." Be sure to encourage the person to give feedback, because besides helping you refine your skills, this will reinforce the point that the patient is an active participant in the Therapeutic Touch process.

After you finish assessing, the person is very likely to ask what you have found. Here again, you must be very careful about your choice of words. In the previous chapter I have used some rather vivid adjectives to help describe subtle energy qualities. *These were for teaching purposes only.* When people are ill, their self-esteem is generally lower than usual and thus they are more psychologically vulnerable. If you tell your patient that you feel a large "void" in such and such a place, you are likely to make him feel worse instead of better! It is both kinder and more helpful to the patient to use words that are as neutral as possible. You can say something like "You need some energy in this area. . . . There is some tightness here. . . . This place needs some balancing. . . ." In this way, you are being honest without adding to the person's anxiety.

It is also important to be careful about your facial expression, which can subtly convey a negative attitude. For example, some beginning practitioners—judging from their expressions—seem to regard the energy congestion as being foul, like sewage, or dangerous, like nuclear waste! A more accurate and helpful point of view is that the congestion is simply a buildup of a natural substance, which, when cleared out of the patient's field, will recycle itself in the environment. If you take this matter-of-fact attitude, it will be reflected in your expression and thus communicated to the patient.

Even though I have emphasized the need for practice,

if you ever get the sense that a person does not really want Therapeutic Touch, you should always respect this attitude and not insist on giving a treatment. Should you try to proceed against your better judgment, you will meet with resistance and the interaction will not be therapeutic. On the other hand, if you yourself do not feel like giving a treatment at a certain time, you should not do it. If someone asks you, you could say, very simply, "I just don't feel up to it today." To be successful, Therapeutic Touch practice must be wholehearted and without reservations; if you have mixed feelings about treating someone, you will be fragmented and the treatment process will not be very effective.

It is possible that when assessing someone for the first time you will not feel anything much at all, even though you know there must be some kind of energy problem because the person is ill and feels miserable. At times like this you can give a general treatment, such as the following:

1) Center yourself and visualize the person as being whole and well.
2) Massage and loosen the person's neck and shoulders.
3) Clear the field once or twice.
4) Hold the feet to stimulate the energy flow and remove tight congestion.
5) Put one hand over the person's solar plexus and the other hand over the kidney area, and direct energy into the person; and then
6) Clear the field again.

When you finish, you can ask the person for feedback. If the reply is, "I feel better except for such and such a place," you can place your hands on the area of discomfort, send energy there, and think of the person as completely well and in balance. Even without a prior assessment, a general treatment such as this can be very helpful. In fact, even if you simply send energy to people, with the intent to help them restore their wholeness, their innate "wisdom of the body" will use the energy appropriately.

Students sometimes ask if any exercises have been designed to improve one's Therapeutic Touch skills. I personally feel that instead of practicing artificially constructed sensitivity exercises, it is more meaningful to use our daily interactions as exercises—that is, to make the way we live in the world consistent with the principles of Therapeutic Touch. For example, since we know that Therapeutic Touch requires an attentive and focused state of mind, we can practice listening to people more attentively, thus achieving a positive feedback between our daily contacts and our treatments.

It is helpful, especially when you are first learning, to give Therapeutic Touch treatments with a partner, because greater insight and understanding can arise out of the interaction between practitioners. However, you and your partner must feel comfortable with each other and be able to cooperate harmoniously. When you work as a team, your individual fields interpenetrate, and thus any discord will interfere with the flow of the energy. The following guidelines should be considered when treating patients together with another practitioner:

1) When assessing, one of you should stand in front of the patient and one in back. Each of you

should pass your hands, side by side, through the patient's field from top to bottom. When the hands of the person in back reach the patient's hips, they should remain there lightly until the partner finishes assessing the patient's legs and feet (see Diagram E). Then you should change places and repeat the procedure. Since the energy flow in front is generally different from that in back, it is important for each of you to assess the whole.

2) It is a good practice, after assessing, to compare your impressions with those of your partner and to decide on an initial plan of treatment. As the patient is an equal participant in the Therapeutic Touch process, be sure to engage her in the discussion. (However, as I mentioned before, be careful about your choice of words.) During the treatment, you should periodically give feedback to one another. Unnecessary talking is a distraction and a hindrance, but feedback about the treatment process is essential.

3) During the treatment it is not necessary for you and your partner to be exactly parallel in your movements; indeed, it is often necessary for one person to work at the patient's head and shoulder area and the other to work at the patient's feet. Each of you, whether in back or in front, should treat appropriately: clear any loose congestion, release any tight areas, and fill in any deficits. As congestion tends to drain downward through the legs, the person in front is responsible for keeping the feet open.

4) At times, you and your partner may want to synchronize your efforts. For example, suppose your patient has an energy blockage that

originates in the spine and extends down through the legs. The person in back could massage the patient's neck and shoulders and send energy down through the entire spinal column. The person in front would stay at the patient's feet throughout the treatment and visualize the healing energy flowing through the spine, down into the legs, out the feet, and into the ground. If you were giving the treatment by yourself, you would first have to treat the spine and then move in front of the patient in order to bring the flow down through the legs and feet. One of the advantages of working with a partner is that all this can be done simultaneously.

5) Most of the time, both practitioners experience the "finished" feeling at the same time. But if one of you finishes before the other, don't walk away. Stay connected with your partner and gently reinforce what she is doing. Remember that your energies and those of your partner are flowing together as a unit, and thus breaking the connection prematurely will disrupt the energy balance and the smooth completion of the treatment.

Because it can be difficult to remain unaffected by the suffering of those we personally love, many students are concerned about treating family members and intimate friends. It would be a shame, however, if we could not use Therapeutic Touch to help those who are closest to us. In such a situation I have found the idea of a hologram[23] to be particularly helpful. Holography is a type of lensless photography performed with laser beams. Any piece of the photographic plate will reconstruct the *entire* image, only in a more blurry form. Various scien-

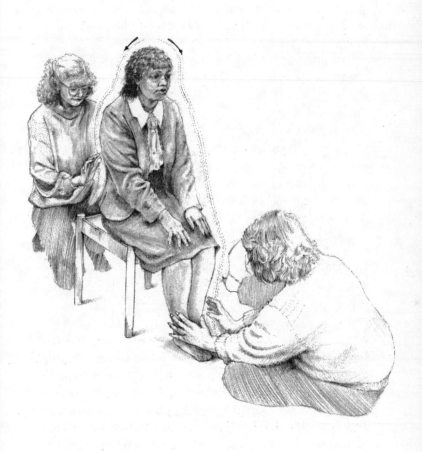

Diagram E: Assessing and Treating with a Partner

tists are now developing theories based on the idea that the universe is essentially a hologram, with every part containing the whole. If we look at humanity as a hologram, then each human being contains, or has access to, the whole human race. Therefore when you treat one person (your sister, your father, your best friend, or even someone you do not particularly like), you are in some mysterious way treating the whole of humanity. I think you will find that if you practice Therapeutic Touch with a holographic attitude—that is, looking upon each patient as a doorway to all humanity—you will be much less likely to lose your center because of your personal feelings toward the individual. Your treatments will also take on a new dimension; they will become universal as well as personal, enriched thereby with a new significance, depth, and beauty.

Carrying this idea further, if we look upon the individual human being as a hologram, then each part of the person somehow contains the whole. It is possible therefore, in these terms, to treat the entire person through an affected part. This approach can be used in emergency situations when there is not time to go through an entire assessment (if, for example, someone falls on the street and sprains an ankle, or burns a finger on the stove) and also whenever a person has to sit or lie in such a way as to prevent you from passing your hands through the entire field (such as a person lying in traction for a back ailment). When you use this approach, however, your intent must be very clear. Even though your hands are holding the affected part, you must always think of helping the essence of the person *through* the part.

Because the energy field is an integrated whole, Therapeutic Touch has been found to be as helpful for those who are emotionally upset as for those who are physically ill. When such people are being treated, however, it is important to stay very calm, for if you should get caught up in the patient's emotional turmoil and find yourself beginning to feel sad, angry, or anxious, the treatment will not be effective. As I mentioned before, emotional as well as vital energy flows throughout the body. For this reason, any emotional upset always has some sort of physical counterpart, the nature of which will, of course, vary with the individual. One person might have a depletion in the stomach, another, tightness in the chest, and so on. Because of this, an emotionally upset individual should be treated in the same manner as anyone else. In addition, you could specifically try to project a feeling of peace and calmness, or visualize the patient filled with blue light.

If the person is upset and confused about some problem, it is important to remember that we ourselves do not have to solve that problem. Our function is to help the person calm down and feel a sense of wholeness so that he can work out a solution or get a better sense of direction. Deep within each person at the intuitive level, there is a resource of creative insight and understanding. We become attuned to this level of consciousness when "our emotions are at peace and our chattering mind is quiet."[24] Thus when we help the patients by calming and balancing their energies, we enable them to achieve, or reconnect with, their own inner sense of direction.

We must also remember that just as emotional problems have physical counterparts, physical problems have emotional counterparts. Thus when you give Therapeutic Touch to someone with a physical problem, the person will respond emotionally as well as physically to the treatment. The most common emotional response is a feeling of quietude and peace. However, emotional tension can be released, and when this occurs the person often starts to cry. If the person cries only a little, you can give some reassurance and continue with the treatment. However, if the crying is intense, stop sending energy, physically touch the person for support, and project a sense of peace and wholeness. Most of the time the crying will stop in a few minutes and the person will feel much better—lighter and more at peace—after this release. Some people will want to talk to you about the problem while others prefer that you sit with them in silence. Use your judgment and do what seems best for the patient. Remember that when treating someone who is releasing emotional tension, or who is emotionally upset, it is essential to remain peaceful and centered. In this way your energy pattern will have a calming effect on the other person, and you will be much less likely to get caught up in his distress.

Since Therapeutic Touch generally has a calming and integrating effect, it can be a helpful adjunct to psychotherapy, especially in times of crisis. However, we have found that psychotic patients, whose sense of self-integrity is so very fragile, often feel violated or intruded upon when we use our hands to help rebalance their energies. The following approach seems to work better with these individuals:

1) Take a deep breath and feel a sense of wholeness within yourself.
2) Keep yourself, physically, a short distance from the person you are going to treat.

3) Visualize the healing energy flowing through the person from the top of the head down through the feet.

4) Think of the person as being well at all levels, in harmony with her essence or sense of inner integrity.

As energy fields permeate space, you can still influence the patient at a distance, but the interaction will not be so intense as to make her feel violated or invaded. Remember, however, to hold firmly to the idea that you are a vehicle for a universal energy. These patients are very fragmented and depleted, and when you open yourself to them they can easily drain you — even at a distance.

Sometimes it is helpful to ask the patient to participate actively in the treatment through visualization. For example, if you are trying to loosen a tight, painful area, the patient can visualize a blue light shining through that particular place. This helps to reinforce what you are doing. There are times, however, when I do not feel it would be appropriate to have the patient participate in this way. If the person, for philosophical or personal reasons, does not believe in the efficacy of visualization, this procedure would be likely to make him feel uncomfortable or artificial. Also, we often forget that visualization requires energy: an effort must be made to focus the mind on a particular image. Therefore, even if a patient believes in visualization (or has at best a skeptical but open-minded attitude) he may be too depleted or tired to do it. It is possible to get around this problem by asking the person to do the exercise for a very short time, say about thirty seconds.

The imagery exercise should be one that is appropriate for the energy problem and also meaningful for the patient. For example, I once treated a young man whose energy field was extremely congested around the area of his abdomen. I suggested that he visualize the healing energy as a light coming down from above, flowing through his abdomen, and going out through his feet. This exercise was appropriate for the particular problem, but it was not meaningful for him. He said that he would rather visualize the energy as a waterfall because to him, water symbolized the flow of universal life. Such experience indicates that instead of assigning someone a specific imagery pattern, it is more helpful to make some suggestions and let the person decide what he prefers.

Sometimes during a treatment you may sense that the person is starting to resist you. This can happen when we are too intense or "heavy-handed." When your sensitivity is not yet fully developed, you may not realize what a definite effect you are having on the patient. Students sometimes think that just because they do not actually feel the energy transfer, nothing is happening. You must remember that the energy will *always* follow your intent, and that the patient is receiving it whether you feel it or not. If you push harder and harder, the patient is likely to feel overwhelmed and/or intruded upon. I have found that many people are quite sensitive to the energy and will react very quickly. Therefore, if you notice that your patient is becoming tense and resistant, *do not push.* Relax, take a deep breath, and try to harmonize yourself with the other person. Proceed very gently. Think of your hands as being as light as feathers and the energy going through them in very fine streams. If the person becomes more tense and irritable, this is probably an indication that she has had enough for the moment.

Students invariably ask, "How often should a person be treated?" The answer, of course, depends on the type of problem and also on the individual. If a relatively healthy person comes home from work with a tension headache or an upset stomach, he will probably need only one treatment. A bad cold or flu should generally be treated every day until the symptoms disappear. An individual who is hospitalized for an acute illness could be treated more than once a day, for a person who is debilitated needs short treatments at frequent intervals. Someone with a chronic or long-term ailment probably should be treated once or twice a week for several months because, as discussed previously, a long-established pattern of ill health generally needs some time to unravel so that a healthier energy pattern can take its place. Even if a patient has a chronic problem, which only manifests or "flares up" at certain times, it is still better to treat the person with some regularity, rather than waiting for the time of an attack. For example, when people with asthma are treated on a regular basis, their attacks become less frequent and less severe. And since their energies are in better balance, a treatment at the time of an attack is more effective than it would have been otherwise.

When you are treating someone every week, it is important to remember that both the quality of each treatment and its results will be somewhat different each time. In my own practice I have noticed that the healing process is generally not a linear one: patients do not usually experience a gradual, day-by-day improvement in their condition. Rather, healing seems to occur in "quantum jumps," or else in a spiraling manner in which short periods of relapse are followed by periods of significant improvement. Many patients are not aware of these normal healing patterns, and unless you reassure them, they can become unnecessarily discouraged when improvement is not noticeable.

After a while you may notice that the treatments begin to have a deeper, more lasting effect. This is a sign that the person is beginning to hold his own, and that you can consider extending the time period between treatments. Many people are sensitive to this change within themselves. One woman recently called me up and said, "I don't need another treatment tomorrow because I'm still processing the one from last week." I was only too happy to reschedule the appointment, because, when all is said and done, this is what we hope for all the patients — the restoration of their wholeness and thus their independence.

5

Self-Transformation Through Therapeutic Touch

The quality of mercy is not strain'd,
It droppeth as the gentle rain from heaven
Upon the place beneath: it is twice bless'd;
It blesseth him that gives and him that takes.

WILLIAM SHAKESPEARE, *The Merchant of Venice*

Many, perhaps most, Therapeutic Touch practitioners feel that they have been changed through the healing process. There is no doubt that the practice of Therapeutic Touch makes us look at the world differently: as a system of flowing energy patterns as opposed to a collection of separate entities. Indeed, when we send the very same vital energy into plants, animals, and human beings, we experience—in a new way—the truth that all life is one life. And with this shift in world view comes a shift in values. It becomes inappropriate to think only of our own betterment, for in an interconnected, dynamic world, the well-being of any individual organism is inseparable from that of all the others.

Since Therapeutic Touch is an interaction, it has the potential to heal the practitioner as well as the patient. Therefore if you give treatments on a regular basis, your own energy field should become more balanced and your health should improve. This is not to say that, as a Therapeutic Touch practitioner, you will never again become ill or upset. That would be an unrealistic expectation because we are all human and we live in a stressful time. However, I think you will find that, as the healing energy flows through you, it will enhance your vitality and sense of well-being.

You can also use the principles of Therapeutic Touch to assist in healing yourself. The practice of this technique indicates that the use of mental imagery can facilitate both the energy transfer and the rebalancing of the patient's field. We also know from biofeedback research that a person can use mental imagery to regulate her physiological processes. Would it not be possible, therefore, for an individual to improve the flow of his *own* vital energy through the use of imagery? Indeed, since the vital energy field is less dense than the physical body, it may prove to be more responsive than the body to conscious repatterning. Many Therapeutic Touch practitioners have successfully experimented with this idea. Right now, if you have pain or discomfort somewhere, you can try it yourself:

1) Sit quietly and center yourself.
2) Visualize the healing energy (as light, if you wish) coming down from above and flowing through you.
3) Visualize the energy clearing away the pain or discomfort (as light shines through a dark area).

To enhance the visualization, you can put your hands over the affected area and see the energy as flowing through your hands, taking the pain away. For a minor problem such as a superficial burn, you may see or feel results fairly quickly; for a serious or chronic problem, however, the visualization exercise would have to be performed on a regular basis for an extended period of time.

Just as the spring rains wash away winter's debris, so the healing energy will clear away the residue of old congestion within your energy field. Therefore, you may at first feel a little stirred up inside, as old tensions (physical and/or emotional) rise to the surface. It is important to remember that these feelings are a residue from the past. Try to observe them in a neutral manner and let them go. If you allow yourself to become caught up in them, they will stay within you, continue to impede your energy flow, and thus damage your health. If an old resentment arises, you can think of it as a cloud being carried away by the wind and disappearing forever. It can also be helpful to talk about it with someone or to write it down in a journal; this serves to objectify the feelings so that they can be released more easily. On the other hand, it is also important not to dwell too much on these old tensions, but to keep your mind involved with the freshness of the present moment. In this way there will be no room within you for old, negative feelings and they will gradually dissipate.

As you practice giving treatments, you will become more and more sensitive to the subtle energy cues that I have been describing. Many practitioners find that this sensitivity cannot be easily turned off at the end of the treatments and that it gradually becomes part of their nature. As a result, you will probably become more sensitive to the energies that surround you wherever you are. You will be more sensitive to beauty and to joy and affection, as well as to ugliness and to sadness and pain. You may want to protect yourself, therefore, when you encounter a situation in which there is a great deal of anger and/or depression. To do this first quiet your mind and then visualize yourself surrounded by the healing energy as a white light. In this way you will not only protect yourself, but you will also influence your environment for the better.

Many practitioners agree that this increased sensitivity directly affects interpersonal relationships. On the one hand, it makes us more aware of the feelings of others and can thus deepen our understanding and empathy. On the other hand, it can cause us to overreact to casual remarks or to issues of minor importance. If you find that this heightened sensitivity is creating difficulties between you and your friends, take some time every day to quiet your mind and attune to your inner center of peace and strength. When we feel calm and secure within ourselves, the things that other people do and say are much less bothersome. If you are having difficulty with a particular individual, you could send this person a thought of peace and wholeness every day. This exercise will help to remove the irritation from your energy field and even affect the other, so that your relationship should improve.

If and when we lose our sense of calmness and integrity during a Therapeutic Touch treatment, it is generally because of some form of attachment to, or over-identification with, one of three aspects of the process: the patient, the results of the treatment, or the role of the practitioner. We tend to over-identify with the patient when that individual is personally significant to us or when his problem is similar to one of our own. Often without realizing it, we feel that the person is an extension of ourselves, so if he is upset we tend to get upset also—a situation that is not at all conducive to healing.

Becoming overly dependent on positive results can also make us lose our balance during Therapeutic Touch. It is perfectly natural to feel that results are important; after all, the purpose of the treatment is to help improve the patient's condition. It is not useful, however, if our sense of self-confidence and self-worth becomes *dependent* on the quality of the results. It is important to remember that we are assisting a highly complex process that essentially takes place *within the patient.* We, personally, are not doing the healing and thus, to a large extent, the type and degree of response is literally "not in our hands." If our sense of inner confidence is dependent on something that is largely out of our control, we are always going to feel insecure and anxious.

I have noticed, from observing myself and others, that we tend to become more concerned and anxious about results if we over-identify with, or become emotionally dependent on, the image of ourselves as "practitioners" or "helpers." When this is the case, we tend to worry about getting positive results in order to justify this self-image. Another effect is that we are in danger of feeling threatened if we ourselves become ill. It is true that if we practice Therapeutic Touch regularly our health may very well improve; but, being human, we do occasionally become ill and need to receive some help ourselves. Therefore, the less we become attached to the "practitioner" image, the freer we are to give and receive through the healing process.

In actual practice the roles of practitioner and patient

are not rigidly separated. I have stressed throughout that Therapeutic Touch is an interaction in which both participants are necessary. In a broad sense, each person is both practitioner and patient: each helps to heal and is healed. The practitioners assist the healing process within the patients and, in doing so, their own level of integration is enhanced; the patients heal themselves through the help of the practitioners, and by participating in this process they help the practitioners' potential to unfold. I have found, in my own practice, that there is a beautiful sense of sharing and equality during Therapeutic Touch. In fact, one person actually said, after her first treatment, "This is more equal than I had thought."

Many students report that it is difficult to avoid being concerned about results when one is a beginner. This is almost inevitable, because feedback is essential when learning something new. Positive feedback—that is, improvement in the patient's condition—tells us that we are using the technique correctly; negative feedback—that is, the patient's discomfort or uneasiness—tells us that something is not right and that we must re-evaluate what we are doing. This information is important and should never be disregarded. Feedback from patients has played an essential role in the development of Therapeutic Touch, and I constantly use this information to modify my own technique. There is a great difference, however, between using feedback—whether positive or negative—to develop our skills and depending on positive feedback to enhance or maintain our sense of self-confidence. It is the latter that creates anxiety and is thus detrimental to the healing process.

Most of us like to feel that we are competent in what we do, and therefore the idea of being a novice or beginner is not very appealing. But herein lies a very important paradox: in order to become more and more competent at Therapeutic Touch, you and I must always be beginners. Learning this method is not accumulating more and more knowledge or information; it is rather a process of allowing a limitless potential to unfold from within. The developmental or learning process itself thus becomes our goal. Thinking that we have achieved a degree of expertise is actually a hindrance because it makes us less open to possibilities for growth. It also tends to make us worry about getting the kinds of results which will justify our expertise. Suzuki-roshi, the Zen master who founded Zen Center in San Francisco, told his students that the goal of practice is always to keep the "beginner's mind."

> In the beginner's mind there is no thought, "I have attained something." All self-centered thoughts limit our vast mind. When we have no thought of achievement, no thought of self, we are true beginners. Then we can really learn something. The beginner's mind is the mind of compassion. When our mind is compassionate, it is boundless. Dogen-zenji, the founder of our school, always emphasized how important it is to resume our boundless original mind. Then we are always true to ourselves, in sympathy with all beings, and can actually practice.[25]

Thus it is best to forget about ourselves, enjoy the process of helping people through Therapeutic Touch, and allow our abilities to unfold spontaneously. Indeed, my colleagues and I have found that the most effective treatments are those in which we are completely absorbed

85

in the healing process itself—a process that is so interesting, so full of wonder and beauty, that it is truly its own reward. Although the practice of Therapeutic Touch is a serious business, it is also a great deal of fun. In a study of adults at play, the researcher Dr. M. Csikszentmihalyi described experiences very similar to those reported by practitioners of Therapeutic Touch: a centering of attention, total involvement and satisfaction in the activity, self-forgetfulness, and spontaneity.[26] In fact, the practice of Therapeutic Touch actually *requires* the present-centered and spontaneous state of being which we associate with play. The patient, as an energy system, is continually changing—both during the treatment and from one treatment to another. The practitioner has to be aware of these changes and respond afresh from moment to moment. It is an exercise in both flexibility and one-pointedness of mind. In our society, work and play are often considered to be separate forms of activity, but in the Therapeutic Touch process we find that the two are integrated.

For most of us, this "totally present," spontaneous attitude or state of inner being arises—paradoxically—out of discipline. Each time we consciously relax and focus ourselves to give a treatment, we repattern or retrain our energy systems to function in a more integrated manner. And as our energies become more integrated, we become more attuned to the subtle voice of the intuition, the faculty through which we perceive patterns and relationships. Our intuition gives us the sense of wholeness: our own wholeness, that of the patients, and the underlying wholeness of the world in which we live. As you learn to trust this inner faculty, it will guide you through all your treatments. Then you will not have to analyze all the details of the process, step by step; on the contrary, you will have an immediate sense of the whole, and your hands — just like those of a sculptor — will simply move to the right places. Each treatment will unfold itself as does a work of art.

Moreover, this intuitiveness will not be limited to your Therapeutic Touch treatments but will begin to permeate all your actions. Many practitioners say that when making decisions, they often have an inner sense of what is right to do — even though, at the moment, they cannot logically explain why. Also, in a broader sense, you will probably become more certain about the direction and the meaning of your life as a whole. For it is this intuitive inner-directedness that gives us our sense of intrinsic identity or completeness as individuals: the sense that we are not living superficially, responding to external pressures alone, but are also in touch with the creative insight of our own inner nature.

True healing, therefore, involves the simultaneous closing of the rifts, or wounds, that exist both within ourselves (between the intuition and the mind, between the mind and the body) and between ourselves and the environment. It involves the realization of our integrity and uniqueness as individuals as well as our unity with the "common life of all which lives."[27] As noted in Chapter 2, this great paradox is inherent in life itself. Every living organism is both a whole and a part, independent and dependent, strong and yet fragile, always the same yet ever-changing. During Therapeutic Touch we can have a deep experience of this paradox, because the healing process involves balancing and strengthening the individual as a whole and also releasing blockages so that he can participate more fully in nature's universal

Notes and References

1. Weber, R., "Philosophical Foundations and Frameworks for Healing," in Kunz, D. (compiler), *Spiritual Aspects of the Healing Arts* (Wheaton, Ill.: Theosophical Publishing House, 1985).
2. *Ibid.*
3. Kunz, D. and Peper, E., "Fields and Their Clinical Implications," in Kunz, *Spiritual Aspects of the Healing Arts.*
4. Jantsch, E., *The Self-Organizing Universe: Scientific and Human Implications of the Emerging Paradigm of Evolution* (Oxford: Pergamon Press, 1980), p. 19.
5. An interesting account of these early days can be found in Krieger, D., *The Therapeutic Touch: How to Use Your Hands to Help or to Heal* (Englewood Cliffs, N.J.: Prentice-Hall, 1979).
6. Krieger, D., "Therapeutic Touch: The Imprimatur of Nursing," *American Journal of Nursing* 75 (1975), 784-87.
7. Grad, B., "Some Biological Effects of the Laying-on of Hands: A Review of Experiments with Animals and Plants,"

Journal of the American Society for Psychical Research 59 (1965), 95-127.

8. Kunz, D., "Dora Kunz Talks About Healing," *Cooperative Connection: Newsletter of the Nurse Healers Professional Associates, Inc.* 1 (1979), 5.

9. A very good discussion of the relationships among relaxation, time perception, and human health can be found in Dossey, L., *Space, Time and Medicine* (Boulder, Colo.: Shambhala Publications, 1982).

10. Krieger, D., *The Therapeutic Touch.*

11. Krieger, D., Peper, E., and Ancoli, S., "Therapeutic Touch: Searching for Evidence of Physiological Change," *American Journal of Nursing* 79 (1979), 660-62.

12. Heidt, P., "Effect of Therapeutic Touch on Anxiety Level of Hospitalized Patients," *Nursing Research* 30 (1981), 32-37.

13. Quinn, J., "Therapeutic Touch as Energy Exchange: Testing the Theory," *Advances in Nursing Science* 6 (1984), 42-49.

14. Bzdek, V. and Keller, E., "Effects of Therapeutic Touch on Tension Headache Pain," *Nursing Research* 35 (1986), 101-6. In this experiment there was a significant difference in pain reduction between the experimental group, which was given Therapeutic Touch, and the control group, which was given a mimic treatment.

15. Weber, R., "Compassion, Rootedness and Detachment: Their Role in Healing. A Conversation with Dora Kunz," in Kunz, *Spiritual Aspects of the Healing Arts.*

16. This issue is discussed in more detail in Briggs, J. and Peat, F. D., *Looking Glass Universe: The Emerging Science of Wholeness* (New York: Simon & Schuster, 1984); and in Weber, R., *Dialogues with Scientists and Sages: The Search for Unity* (London: Routledge and Kegan Paul, 1986).

17. Kunz, F. L., "The Reality of the Non-material," *Main Currents in Modern Thought* 32 (Retrospective Issue, 1940-75), 16-23. See also Weber, *Dialogues with Scientists and Sages,* pp. ix-xi.

18. Kunz, D. and Peper, E., "Fields and Their Clinical Implications," p. 215.

19. Quinn, J., "Therapeutic Touch as Energy Exchange: Testing the Theory."

20. A detailed description of this process, from the energy field perspective, can be found in Kunz and Peper, "Fields and Their Clinical Implications," Part 1.
21. Saint-Exupéry, A., *Wind, Sand and Stars* (New York: Harcourt, Brace & World, 1940), p. 66.
22. Feng, Gia-Fu and English, J. (trans.), *Tao Te Ching* by Lao Tsu (New York: Alfred A. Knopf, 1972).
23. For more information, see Wilber, K. (ed.), *The Holographic Paradigm and Other Paradoxes* (Boulder, Colo.: Shambhala Publications, 1982).
24. Kunz and Peper, "Fields and Their Clinical Implications," p. 222.
25. Suzuki, Shunryu, *Zen Mind, Beginner's Mind* (New York: John Weatherhill, 1970), p. 22.
26. Csikszentmihalyi, M., "Play and Intrinsic Rewards," *Journal of Humanistic Psychology* 15 (1975), 41-63.
27. Arnold, E. (trans.), *The Song Celestial: A Poetic Version of the Bhagavad Gita* (Wheaton, Ill.: Theosophical Publishing House, 1975), p. 41.

ARKANA – NEW-AGE BOOKS FOR MIND, BODY AND SPIRIT

A selection of titles

With over 200 titles currently in print, Arkana is the leading name in quality new-age books for mind, body and spirit. Arkana encompasses the spirituality of both East and West, ancient and new, in fiction and non-fiction. A vast range of interests is covered, including Psychology and Transformation, Health, Science and Mysticism, Women's Spirituality and Astrology.

If you would like a catalogue of Arkana books, please write to:

Arkana Marketing Department
Penguin Books Ltd
27 Wright's Lane
London W8 5TZ